THE BBL BIBLE:

How to get a butt to die for,
without dying for it

Dr. Scott Blyer aka DrBfixin ⚒

Medical Director of Cameo Surgery

The BBL Bible: How to get a butt to die for without dying for it
Copyright © 2020 Scott Blyer, MD
All rights reserved. No portion of this book may be reproduced in any form without permission from the publisher, except as permitted by U.S. copyright law.

For information about this title or to order books contact
drb@cameosurgery.com

This book is not intended as a substitute for the medical advice of physicians. the reader should regularly consult a physician in matters relating to his/her health.

Print ISBN: 9781734414905
Printed in the United States of America

Dedication

I've read hundreds of book, maybe even thousands and the dedication section usually looks the same.

People dedicated their book to their spouse or kids, and I wondered, why are they all the same? Is there no one else to dedicate this to?

This morning, as I write this at 4:30 am on Sunday, I finally get it. I started this book over 2 years ago and have been dragging my ass on it. Trying to find time for this has been in early mornings, late nights, and weekends. Over this time, I consistently have whined, "I gotta finish the book", been falling asleep at the dinner table and have a hundred other unfinished projects that has taken a back seat to this.

So for this reason, I dedicate this book to my beautiful wife and my delicious daughter, and apologize for complaining for the last two years and appreciate their patience. Now I can clean the garage.

To the haters, you have made me elevate my game and want to work even harder. So thanks.

I thank the patients who have trusted me to care for them, and my team for always believing in the DrBfixin way of life. We are different, no doubt, and it takes courage to be different.

Behind all of my daily activities I am inspired by the teaching of both of my parents. I love you both. Although my mom is isn't physically here to pick up the phone, or share in the wins and losses, she has given me the compass to figure shit out. I hope I have made you proud.

Foreword

Some books must be read knowing about the author's bias. I got none. No none gives me free shit. I don't have any financial stake in any company I write about, aside from my own business. This book is written with no bullshit. This is the honest truth, with no crap. This book wasn't written to sell machines, or sell me as a doctor. It was written to educate you on real talk with regard to the BBL surgery. It may not be for you, but at least you have the information to decide for yourself, no cap.

This book is written in a language that is meant to be easily read and understandable. Some people may find my style offensive because everyone is so sensitive nowadays. For those people, maybe you can return this book before it's too late. At no point did I want to write something to gas myself up on how smart I am. This was not written for ego. In fact any medical word that could be confusing I tried to explain in simple terms. It wasn't written to make money. It cost a lot to print this shit in color. I really wrote this to help you make decisions, save some lives, and give you the best results after this life changing surgery. Enjoy. Stay fixin my friends,

DrBfixin

Table of Contents

Dedication	3
Foreword	5
Chapter 1: Wish pics	11
Chapter 2: I want that ass	20
Chapter 3: I need more sauce.	26
Chapter 4: Will My Skin Be Loose?	33
Chapter 5: Cellulite and weird skin on the ass	45
Chapter 6: BBL after massive weight loss	53
Chapter 7: BMI (whats the deal?)	62
Chapter 8: Multiple surgeries at the same time?	67
Chapter 9: Choosing your doctor	72
Chapter 10: Price	78
Chapter 11: Do you get what you pay for?	83
Chapter 12: It's cheaper in other countries	86
Chapter 12: Alternatives to fat	93
Chapter 13: Silicone butt implants	105
Chapter 14: Butt Shots: Everything you want to know, and everything your NEED to know	111
Chapter 15: The FDA and their 'approval'	122
Chapter 16: Getting ready for surgery, and the perfect candidate	129
Chapter 17: Anesthesia options	132
Chapter 18: Liposuction techniques	139
Chapter 19: Hemoglobin and anemia - who cares?	147
Chapter 20: What is the deal with these embolisms?	156

Chapter 21: Is it Safe?	163
Chapter 22: Ultrasound assisted BBL (the safest way to do a BBL -in my opinion)	182
Chapter 23: My recipe for a successful and safe technique	186
Chapter 24: Complications	189
Chapter 25: What to expect day 1 and early on	213
Chapter 26: Going to the bathroom	221
Chapter 27: Sitting	227
Chapter 28: Sleeping	232
Chapter 29: Eating	237
Chapter 30: Showering	241
Chapter 31: Cleaning the faja	243
Chapter 32: I'm gonna faint!	245
Chapter 33: Garments	248
Chapter 34: Lymphatic Massages	260
Chapter 35: Pain	269
Chapter 36: More patient feedback	276
Chapter 37: Exercising	277
Chapter 38: Incisions and secret tips	280
Chapter 39: What do I put on my scars?	292
Chapter 40: Shit people will try to sell you that's bullshit	299
Chapter 41: Waist trainers	309
Chapter 42: The Art of the Twerk	320
Chapter 43: Excuses you can use if you wanna lie	328

Chapter 44: Haters	330
Chapter 45: FAQ	334
Chapter 46: The future	337
About the author:	343

Chapter 1: Wish pics

"Ass so big, I told her to look back at it"
                                    2 Chainz

Ass is life. The world's growing addiction to a nice fat ass has pushed the Brazilian Butt Lift to higher heights. We, as doctors, essentially create designer butts. Instagram models and popular reality stars have become the icons and wish pics for many of our patients. These wish pics if used correctly can be an amazing tool for the doctor and patient.

Subjective words traditionally used when planning a surgery, like "natural looking", or "not too crazy" can mean different things to each party. Patients have told me, I want a natural looking booty and I ask them to show me one on IG. Then they pull up a picture of a monstrous ass. You as a patient should bring some photos of butts that not only you like, but what you think is achievable with your body. Ahh, there is the rub…

That is where these pictures can be a bad thing. So many of these pictures on IG are photoshopped and is terribly misleading. I would like to think doctor's pages are more ethically sound and they do not photoshop pictures on their page. I will say most do not photoshop, however I know some do. Shame on you. There are subtle things the trained eye may pick up in the photo that are the giveaway, but some people are very good with the available apps and editing software where it can be essentially undetectable (ask Kim).

Then there are other photos that are not photoshopped but they have very exaggerated results from other non recommended procedures, such as silicone injections, or rib removal. We have had IG models who look gorgeous on their page, come in with major problems from bad decisions they made earlier in the career. Just because it looks good in a picture doesn't mean it is not hard as a rock, loaded with nodules, and causes pain for them. Injectable liquid silicone is dangerous and illegal and will be covered more extensively later in the book (Chapter 14). The beauty of silicone is it flows through tissue incredibly smoothly and easily when it is injected. That is why it is injected into tight tethered down acne scars and behind the eyeball to treat retinal detachments. It can fill a tight butt gorgeously which will look amazing in photos, but in real life it can be rock hard, lumpy, cystic, migrate to other areas and spots of necrosis (dead butt tissue) can be evident. I have neither met Bernice Burgos, nor felt her ass :(but, by her own admission in an interview she explained she had such injections in a Bronx basement. Silicone is a dangerous chemical that has no business being injected into a butt, but it is tempting for many girls. It looks good, it is cheap, and look how successful someone like Bernice has become. I'm sure she's a wonderful person but I think her body has a lot to do with it. She is the wish pic of so many of my patients.

In these booty forums people have non medical terms like hip dips and laterals that aren't accepted medical terminology and if your doctor isn't lit like me, (lol, really though) he may have no idea what you are referring to. Photos are worth a thousand words.

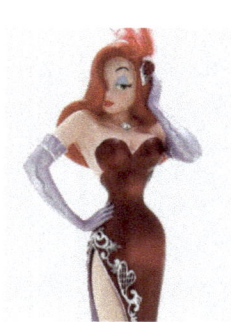

Men have an innate preference for

female bodies with narrow waists and full hips, which signal high fertility, high estrogen, and low testosterone. Even cartoon characters are rocking big asses. Females like Jessica Rabbit, Lara Croft, and ElastiGirl from the Incredibles all have exaggerated proportions.

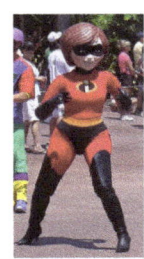

When people discuss waist to hip proportions they are referring to the diagram to right:

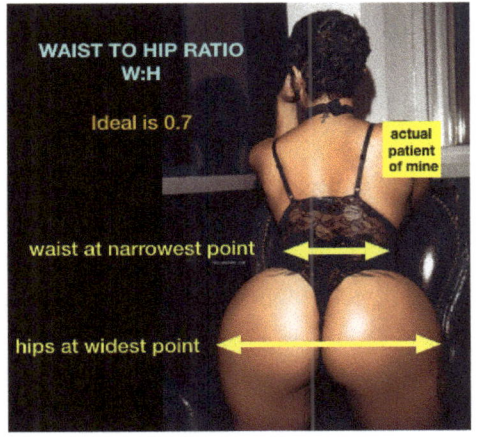

During the twentieth century, Miss Americas' and Playboy Centerfolds' waist-to-hip ratios ranged from 0.68 to 0.72. In 2016 a survey was performed with several thousand plastic surgeons revealing a new ideal waist to hip ratio of 0.6 and 0.65 was the trend. More recently another was study was in the Journal of Plastic and Reconstructive Surgery showing a newer ideal ratio of 0.7.

Surgeons in their 40s and the younger general population in their 20s liked proportionally larger butts. That same study showed Latin American male surgeons had a preference for the largest butts.

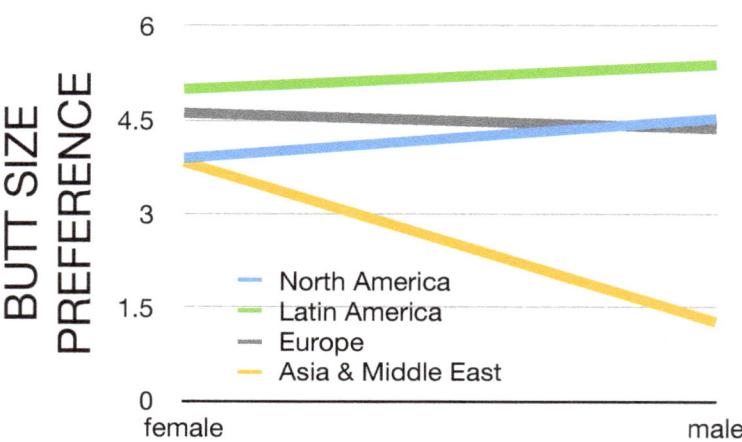

Beauty is subjective. Look at some of the couples you know that don't look like they belong together. Something we can agree upon is the human eye likes continuity and balance, even moreso than symmetry. Bigger butts are definitely in vogue and looks popping, but I personally do not like it when it doesn't flow well with the legs. Many of my patients refer to this mismatch as "ant ass" or "diaper ass".

The butt shape is determined mostly biologically. Namely the position, shape and size of your pelvis and the distribution of fat and muscle in this area. Obviously a person's weight contributes to the shape as does their musculature, for those that do or do not put in time for those squats. It is often best to go with what your body is naturally shaped for. Ironically, whether patients realize or not, most patients do request the shape that is consistent with the shape of their body-just bigger.

Women generally come in with one of these four shaped butts.

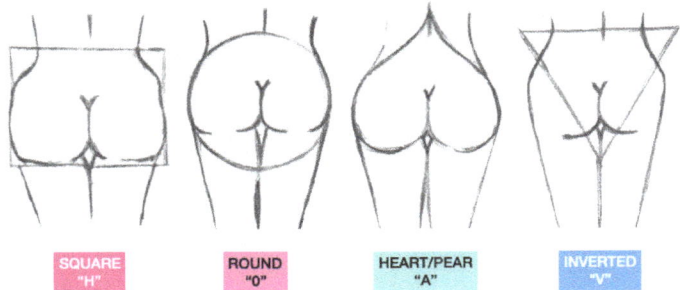

The square butt: These people often refer to themselves as sponge bob asses. This shape is a little more masculine in style and are flat across the bottom and sometimes even prolapsed a little (with a bulge in the lower portion, closest to the butt crack). People generally do not ask for this shape. It often a magnified by a lack of fat in the hips.

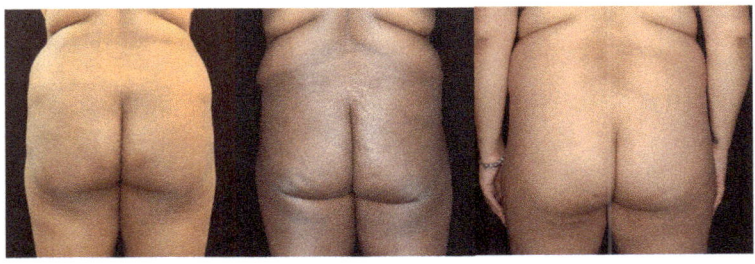

The round butt: often called the bubble butt. This is a round circular shape and has an athletic look to it.
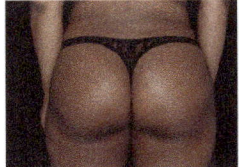
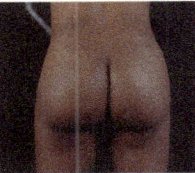
I refer this as the volleyball butt.

The upside down heart butt: this is also called the pear shaped butt. It has a tapered look from the top to the bottom. It is a very feminine shape with fullness in the areas of deficiency of the inverted V butt.

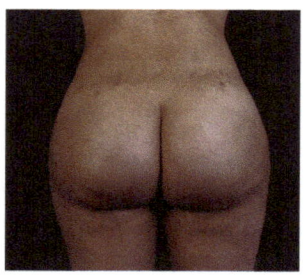

The inverted V: This butt can be so inverted it looks like an arrowhead. This butt shape is fuller on top but on the lower lateral portions (outside positions), it is under developed. On the right butt cheek this is at 4 and 5 o'clock and on the left 8 and 7 o'clock positions. It is the complete opposite of the upside down heart butt. It is a right side up heart.

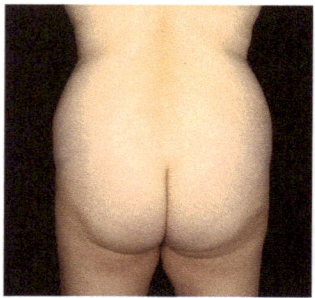 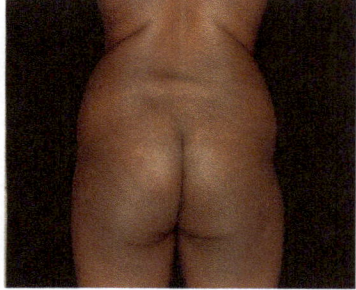

The two most common requested booty shape is the upside-down heart (or pear), followed by the round (volleyball) butt.

In my opinion if you have an upside down heart shaped butt or a round butt it is best to go with it and enhance that shape and style. If you have a square butt or an inverted

V, the best shape for you should be made on a case by case basis with you and your surgeon.

As important as the butt is, almost equally important are the hips. So many people bring me BBL wish pics and they are front photos where you do not even see the back view. I personally dislike overly done hips that make a patient look like a centaur [1].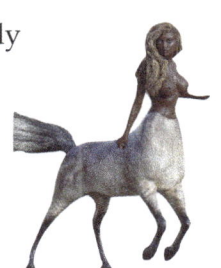

There are certainly cultural and ethnic differences in what is deemed attractive for the butt. With regard to projection it generally seems as African-Americans like the highest point of projection, Caucasians in the middle, and Hispanics generally like it lower.

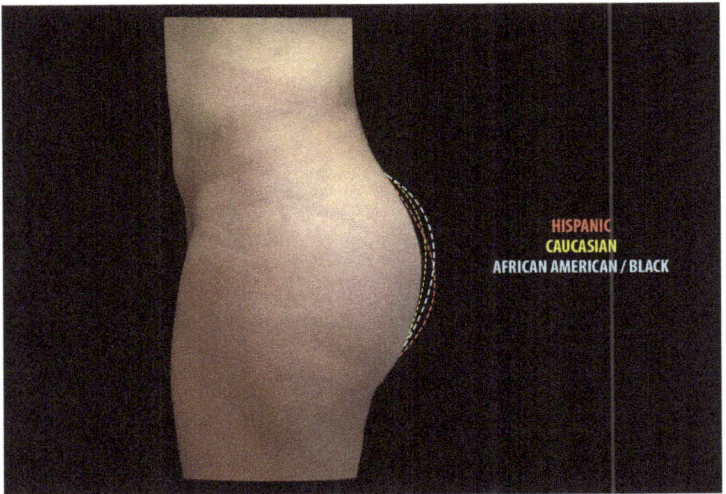

---

[1] centaur - is a mythological creature from Greek mythology with the upper body of a human and the lower body and legs of a horse.

Sometimes a Caucasian patient is in a relationship with a Black man and/or hangs out with Black people and identifies characteristics of an African American butt more attractive. For this reason it is important to talk to the patient about what they like and what they can get according to their shape and vice versa.

In summary, wish pics are a double edge sword. It helps the patient get their ideas across to the doctor which is great. The pictures chosen however, may not be authentic and have been modified. If it was unaltered, it may not have been achieved with a fat transfer alone, or it may have taken multiple rounds of surgery. As long as a patient understands this before surgery, mission accomplished. And finally, we cannot change someones physical makeup. If you have always been a larger woman with a high body mass index, if it impossible to make you into a petite flower in a simple surgical procedure. This is not a reflection of the skill of the doctor, it is just a fact. Our bodies change as we mature. Bringing in a picture of your body at age 18 and coming to the office at 50 after 4 kids, it will be far fetched to believe turning back the clock to that teenage body is possible.

As for men, a conversation must be had with regard to the look they are going for. Most men want a more muscular shaped butt that looks like muscle.. Some men want a rounded feminine butt. In my experience it seems as though fat added to the butt of a man tends to survive more than that of a female. This may be due to a generally larger muscle and therefore better blood supply to the butt. .

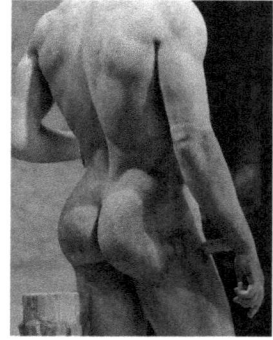

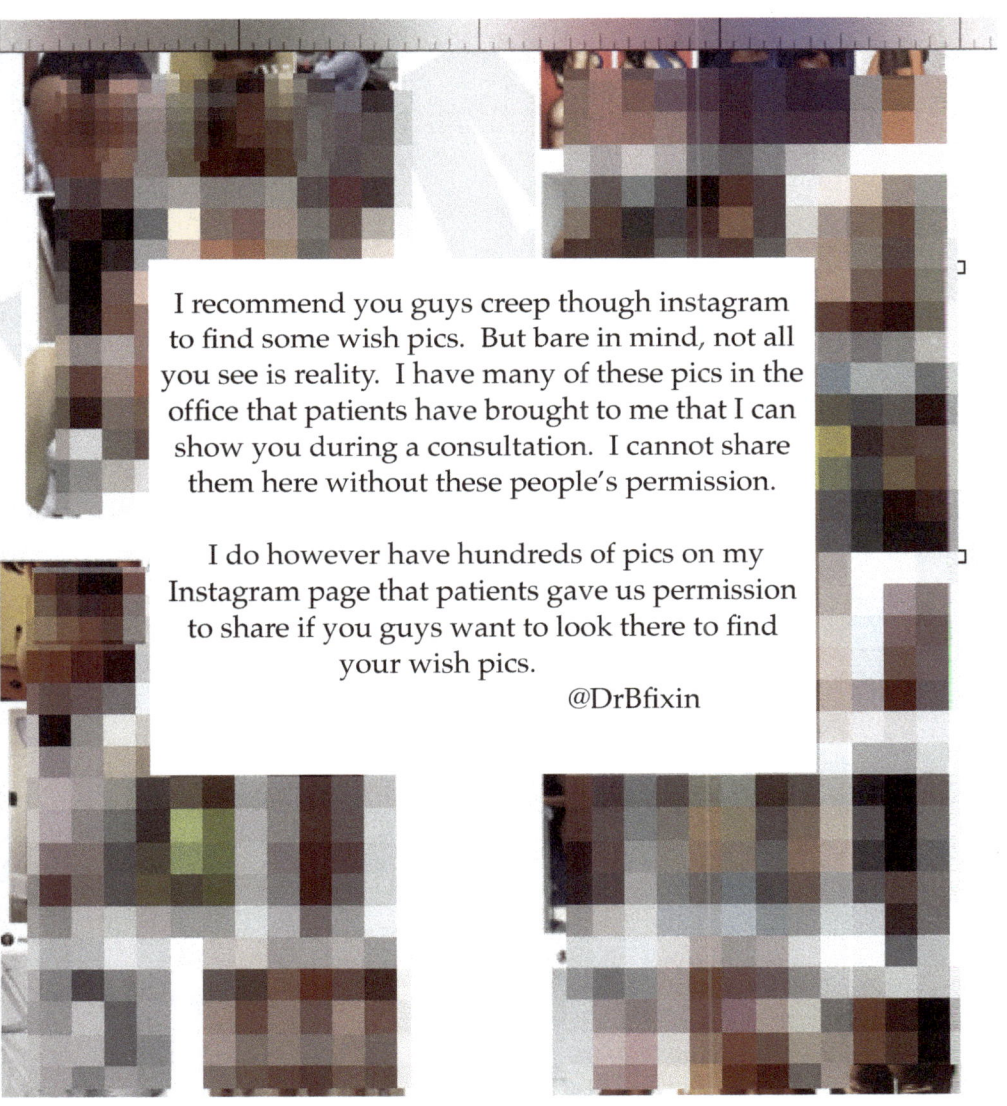

I recommend you guys creep though instagram to find some wish pics. But bare in mind, not all you see is reality. I have many of these pics in the office that patients have brought to me that I can show you during a consultation. I cannot share them here without these people's permission.

I do however have hundreds of pics on my Instagram page that patients gave us permission to share if you guys want to look there to find your wish pics.

@DrBfixin

Chapter 2: I want that ass

"Oh my God Becky? Look at her butt!"
Lil Wayne

The two things that limit how large we can create a butt is:
1. Do we have enough fat?
2. Will the skin stretch enough to fit the fat?

On the average it is believed that 30% of the fat that is injected is lost. It is for that reason it is best to overfill the butt, and to believe when you leave the office you should think your butt looks a little too big. It is very rare to have a butt end up larger than the patient wants. There are very few complaints after surgery in my practice. **If** our patients have any complaints about the size after surgery, 99% of the complaints are I wish it was a little bigger.

Everyone has different booty goals and one's conception of a big enough butt varies from individual to individual. Everyone wants a snatched waist. Most people want a belly that's flat flat. There are some that like slim thick. The booty and hips however is quite variable and was covered in the previous chapter.

Looking back at our best booty before and after results, I have seen the perfect balance of enough fat but not too much fat is a BMI of 26-28. The BMI is a calculation based on height and weight (more about BMI in Chapter 7). As long as the BMI is in that range, and one's booty goals are reasonable, there should be enough fat to make the butt you desire.

The next issue is will the skin stretch enough to fit the fat I want. Some butts are tighter than others. This goes for the hips too. People that lose a lot of weight or has stretch marks on their butt usually, but not always, will stretch enough. Normally when you grab some skin, the pinch of skin follows the arch of the pinch.

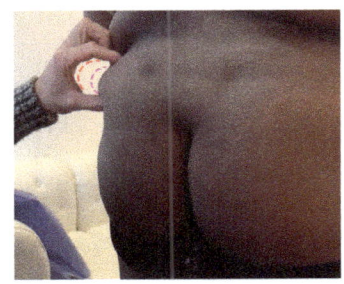

There are some butts that have areas that fail to follow a smooth arc, When looking carefully at photos there are also patients with underdeveloped areas of the butt which present with an internal band that prevents the skin from expanding.

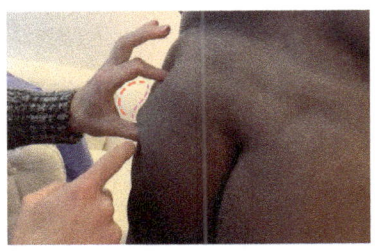

Sometimes these tight areas can be seen on an ultrasound. Please take note of how normals areas of the butt have nice clearly defined fascial layers separating the fat of the butt into two broad general compartments. In a constricted area you can see that there are multiple overlapping layers of fibrous tissue not allowing the skin to smoothly stretch and release out (picture on right).

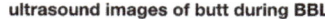
ultrasound images of butt during BBL

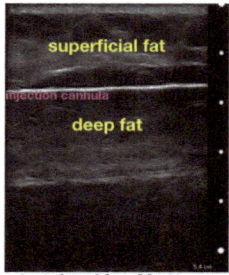
superficial fat
deep fat

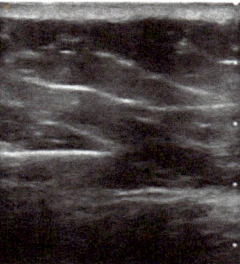

stretchy skin of butt: nice and clean sections

tight area of butt: many layers of fibers holding skin down

If these tight stubborn areas are encountered during surgery, trying to overpower the area by multiple passes trying to release the bands can result in a very unfavorable outcome. There is more about this situation in the chapter covering complications (Chapter 24). It is best to either remove the fat above it to camouflage the area and make the 'peak above the band' or leave it as is and allow the skin to stretch. It can be revisited in 3 months and a touch up can be done. By adding a small amount of fat later, the skin had a chance to stretch and is more likely to accommodate the extra fat. There are some who are still resistant to this, and the limit to what can be accomplished may have already been reached.

It is best to point this out to the patient before the surgery. These internal band will prevent the skin from stretching to a nice dome shape.

Started from the bottom now we here.
The bottom 'cuff' of the butt is referred to as the inferior (lower)

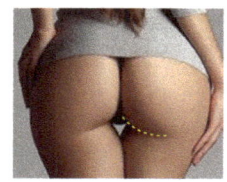

gluteal fold.   Many people find the short gluteal crease attractive.
 This area caries quite a bit patient to patient..
The fold may appear very short.
The fold may appear quite long.

They may appear at a different heights.

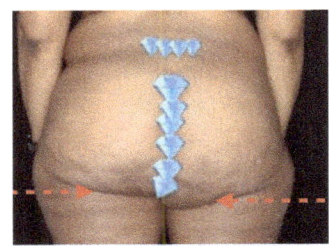

folds are different heights

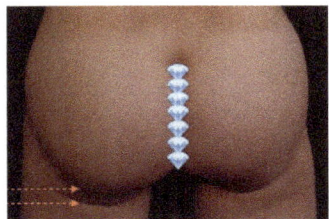

Some people have a double fold under the butt.

Others may have a small pedunculated area that hangs lower than the rest of the fold that gives the appears of a wavy crease. It can accentuate the square shape of a butt and can be corrected with some lipo.

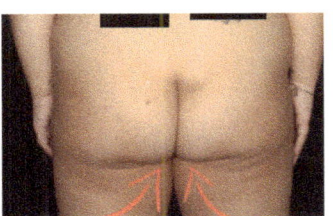

Almost everyone wants a scooped out back. **This is a created by multiple factors:**

- **fat**
    - this is something that we   **In the doctor's control**

23

generally remove with liposuction

- **skin adherence to the deeper tissue**
    - sometimes an incision may be needed to make the skin envelope tighter in these spots, other times good compression in that spot after lipo, or even j plasma skin tightening may help, and in some patients this area cannot be improved

    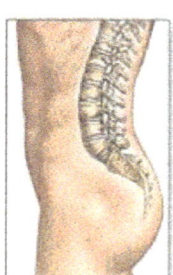 sometimes in the doctor's control

- **spinal curve**
    - this is called lordosis and is actually spinal curvature. It is common in dancers gymnasts and certain conditions can contribute to lordosis. Imbalances in muscle strength and length are also a cause, such as weak hamstrings, or tight hip flexors. It is actually bad for your spinal health in the long term, but it makes your booty pop in the short term.

    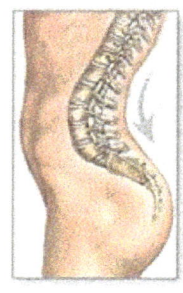

    Lordosis of the spine — Exaggerated lumbar curve

    Normal spine

    ✘ not in the doctor's control

- **posture at the time of that selfie**
    - it amazes me how much some of these girls can pop that booty out when it's time for that photo.

    ✓ In the doctor's control

- **how good you are with Facetune.** not everything is as it appears in pictures. They did it for the gram.

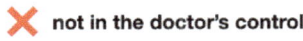 not in the doctor's control

Unfortunately there are situations when the patient knows what they want. The doctor knows what the patient wants and he/she wants it too. However, the anatomy does not cooperate. It is best to identify these potential problems before surgery so it becomes a warning, rather than noticing it later when it becomes an excuse. It is a collaborative agreement. The doctor has to be the guide, and identify and properly explain these problems to the patient so they can understand. The patient has to hear and be willing to listen (not the same thing) and trust the experience of the doctor so they won't be disappointed later.

Chapter 3: I need more sauce.
How to gain weight, and what if I loose weight?

"Draw me a rainbow. Here is a pencil."
Laura Lana Lane Bidegain Spinelli 3 M Katherine Nice, 2019

Do I have enough fat is a question I am asked daily. And believe it or not, the next common question I get is, "How do I gain weight"? My friends reading this with a BMI of 33 and above are rolling their eyes right now (me too, lol).

The amount of fat you need is entirely based on what your booty goals are. Are you looking for that Black Chyna, music video vixen ass or are we going for a humble athletic one, or the corporate booty. The next consideration is what are you starting with. Do you have nothing back there? Are you so far from your dream booty that you will likely need two visits?

Most butts can tolerate up to up to 2400 cc of fat without looking distorted. At some point there is a limit to how much the skin will stretch without losing its round shape.

For those that want a natural shaped butt with nice curves and projection the amount of fat needed is a BMI of 25-28. If you are looking for a large kapoooow butt you may need more. The most fat I have been able to fit in someone's butt and still have a nice result is 3500 cc. When too much is injected the roundness of the butt becomes distorted and the fat will literally shoot out of the hole in which it is being injected from.

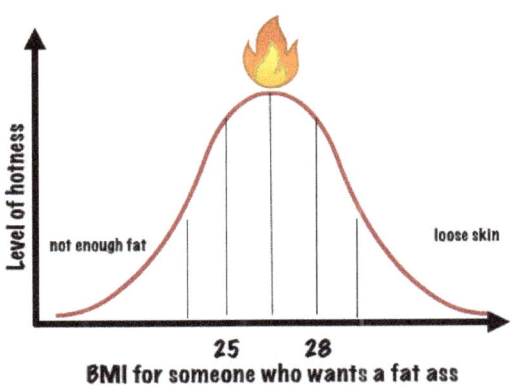

If you are looking for that music video butt you may need to return for a second surgery, and even a third surgery depending on your goals.

I cannot gain weight, what do I do?
Well, boo hoo hoo. Just kidding. We do have a lot of patients with this 'problem'. We encourage people who need to gain weight to do everything they were always told not to do. Eat before bed. Drink your calories. We have had patients find success in going to Vitamin Shoppe or GNC and getting weight gaining shakes that body builders use. I would drink 1-2 of these per day. Especially one before bed, when your metabolism is slow.

The downside of this is we cannot obviously control where the fat will go. Some people are prone to gaining visceral fat. That is fat under the abdominal muscles that is not accessible during lipo. This is many times seen in people after who gain weight after lipo or a tummy tuck. Some people gain it in their legs, face, or arms. Just be prepared that you may want to 'add on' another spot if you were planning on doing lipo 360 than you get fat in your arms instead. If you gain enough weight, eventually it should spill over to the areas that were part of the plan. If may even go to your butt!

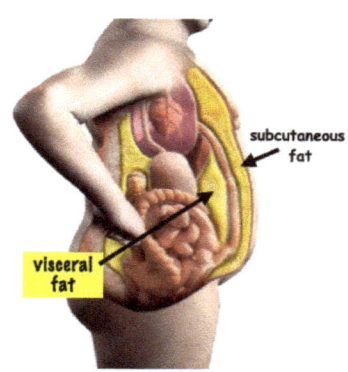

What if I lose weight after surgery?

Fat in the body is essentially all white fat. Brown fat is found predominantly in newborns and decreases as we age. It can be found in random areas like around the spinal cord and shoulder blades.

Even though the majority of fat in the body is white fat, fat has different behavior depending on where it is located in the body. For example for fat transfers to the face where a little fat is needed, knee fat is excellent as a source for harvesting. Knee fat is very resilient fat. Fat from different areas of the body maintain their characteristics despite where they are moved to. So fat from the knee injected into the face, is knee fat that now lives in the face.
So we try to remove stubborn areas of fat during liposuction. This is fat that no matter how much you diet and exercise, is still there. Therefore, when we inject this

fat into the butt, it is now stubborn fat that no matter how much you diet and exercise lives in the butt.

We recommend at least maintaining your weight or losing just a little. If you loose a tremendous amount of weight, it will start to come off your butt.

What if I gain weight after surgery?
The initial gain in fat will go to the areas where the majority of your fat cells live, your butt. At some point it will spill into other areas as well.

I thought once you get lipo I cannot get fat in that area again?
This is not true. Fat cells are microscopic and not every fat cell can be removed.

It is true that this will likely not be the first place the fat will go. It will go to the place where the majority of fat resides. Your belly can get fat even after lipo of the belly, but much of it can become visceral fat. Again, this is deep fat

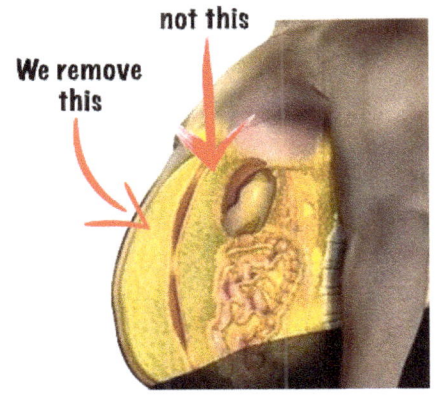

that protects your internal organs that cannot be removed without weight loss and exercise.

The difference between subcutaneous fat and visceral fat

subcutaneous fat	visceral fat
superficial, under the skin	deep, under the muscle
pinchable	cannot be pinched, bulge
soft	firm
lipo, non surgical fat reduction treatments, diet, exercise can decrease	diet, and exercise only can decrease

There was a theory being pushed by doctors known as the 'fat distribution theory', that we have a certain number of fat cells in our body and if they are removed, your body will have memory of it and reform them elsewhere. This has been proven to be incorrect. If you gain weight after lipo, the fat that was permanently removed is still permanently removed. You may gain size in the untreated areas, or the areas that were the recipient of the fat transfer (your butt).

Can I take fat from someone else?
So many people ask me this. I think some are joking but I am certain a few of them truly mean it. Imagine getting an organ donation from someone else. This person must be a 'match' of blood type and cross matching tissue compatibility. The recipient is often a lifelong slave to taking steroids and anti rejection medications which had lower your immune system and increase your risk of

cancer. Organ transplants are performed as non elective surgery that is life saving.

While a nice ass can be relationship saving, it is hard to imagine the medical community being ok with this as an option. The recipient could theoretically acquire any blood borne disease from the donor including but not limited to HIV, Hepatitis, or even an occult cancer, if microscopic cancer cells were transferred. Jacoby and Meyers would be all over this one!

That being said, it has been done in California from mother to daughter for post breast cancer reconstruction, and has been successful. It has been done in Korea with a larger group of women with no major complications. In this litigious country we live in, where people will sue anyone for anything, and some blood sucking lawyer would take just about any case, I do not think any sane doctors would take on the responsibly and exposure of these risks. It is not recommended.

Will my breasts be bigger after lipo?
Studies have looked at this and lipo will not increase the size of your breasts. Your breasts may appear larger in proportion to a smaller frame, and if you gain weight your breasts may get larger but the lost fat cells will not cause more fat cells to grow in your breasts.

Are there any health benefits to liposuction?
Intuitively one would think that cholesterol levels and or diabetes should improve after liposuction. This has not

proven to be the case in the medical literature. If someone is thinner, perhaps they will have an easier time to exercise and more motivated to get started with an exercise regiment but there is no direct correlation with ones' health. That being said, if someone's confidence is improved they are less likely to suffer from depression. People who are more attractive receive more attention in school, have better marriages, make more money, and get more personalized attention. These facts have been shown in the medical literature.

Chapter 4: Will My Skin Be Loose?

"Oh, Rump-o'-smooth-skin, you say you wanna get in my Benz?"

Sir Mix A Lot

Skin thickness is low key one of the most important features of the predictability of the skin to retract after liposuction, but no one really talks about it. Different areas of the body have different thicknesses of skin. The lower eyelids has the thinest areas which measures 0.5 mm in depth, and the heel of the foot is can be 8 times thicker.

Why is this so important? Think of it this way. If you put a brick on your bed and cover it with a thick down comforter you would not even know the brick is there. However, if you put a brick on your bed and covered the brick with a thin top sheet instead of the comforter, you would see the outline of the brick very well. In this example, the skin is represented by the comforter (thick skin) or top sheet (thin skin). This is very important and usually addressed by rhinoplasty surgeons before doing a nose job. Usually the patient with a thick bulbous nasal tip will have a hard time ever achieving a look of a thin tip because of the skin thickness, something that cannot be altered too much (it can be thinned a little in the nose, but that is not what this book is about).

It is also important in liposuction. Those with thick skin is great for liposuction for the surgeon. It hides irregularities and lumps and bumps very well. A thin skinned patient is more likely to see the indentations from the cannula passes. The liposuction cannulas used are between 3-5 mm in diameter and are shaped like thin sticks with suction holes at the end. Thicker skin is more likely to retract as well. That doesn't mean if you are removing a large amount of fat it will be super tight. It means it will retract better than a thin skinned person.

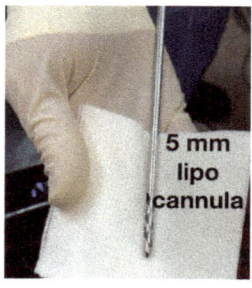

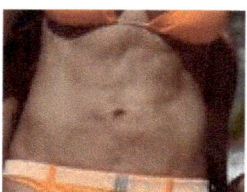

Other indictors of poor skin elasticity include:
- stretch marks on the skin
- women who gave birth to a child
- women who gave birth to multiple children
- people who lost a significant amount of weight
- someone who is overweight with skin that can be pinched more than 1 inch
- genetic predisposition
- smokers
- post menopausal women
- people who had massive weight loss surgery
- people over the age of 35

Generally the back has thicker skin than the abdomen. Perhaps we have evolved to have thicker skin on our back for carrying heavy loads, or sleeping on our back, or some more protection, whatever the case may be, we have thicker skin on our back. Additionally, it is less likely to show indents from lipo. There are situations that a patient will come to my office telling me that they have had liposuction twice on their back elsewhere, and they are still

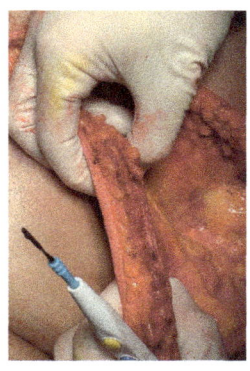

fat. Many times this is just the thick skin that remains. These people will grab what they perceive as back fat and claim they have fat in their back. Shown in the picture to the left is the thickness of the skin on the back between my fingers. Now multiply it by two, by folding that skin on itself

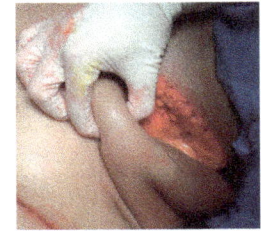

and it feels even thicker (picture on right). While the skin can shrink a little on the back after lipo and whatever other skin tightening modalities you want to perform with it (j plasma or laser lipo), the rolls will remain. The sure way to remove them is a bra lift. Most offices call it an upper body lift. This is a scar across the back under the bra strap. Sometimes it is straight across sometimes a small gap of skin can be left between the right and left sides.

Abdominoplasties (tummy tucks) have become commonplace and generally accepted as a necessity to a flat stomach. Just like the skin of the belly stretches when someone gains fat on their belly, the skin on the back also stretches to accommodate the fat.

Have I seen people have loose skin after lipo when I was not expecting it? Rarely, but it has happened. It is more likely in light skinned people and when the post operative garment is too tight. I had a young patient without children who was not overweight who I anticipated would have a nice result. I placed her in the appropriate garment and she returned in two weeks wearing a waist trainer. Her skin was now damaged and although her butt looked incredible she had some loose skin that we both were not expecting as a result of her wearing the wrong garment provided by her friend, ignoring my advice.

If you are warned by your doctor that will have loose skin and you are choosing not to have a skin reduction surgery (tummy tuck, bra lift, etc) you are best wearing a loose garment. Allow it to gently place the skin in the proper position. Pull the skin up in the front. Do not allow for the skin to hang over your underwear. This technique is just like when a woman pulls her breasts up in a bra. Put on the garment and once it's closed, slide your hand down the front and pull the skin up. A piece of foam can be helpful keeping the skin up.

Nature does the best job at allowing for the skin to retract. By the patient wearing a garment too tight it is actually counter productive and will not allow the skin retract nicely. Picture how much a belly stretches to accommodate a baby. The skin retracts by a process called apoptosis. Wearing something too tight will not allow the skin to heal properly.

Skin retracts very well in the arm. Skin retracts very poorly in the inner thigh area.

For those we anticipate will have loose skin
The Ehlers-Danlos syndromes (EDS) are a group of related disorders caused by different genetic defects resulting in poor collagen strength. The primary complications seen in EDS involve the skin, muscles, skeleton, and blood vessels. Patients with EDS often have skin that can be describes as "velvety", "loose". This skin characteristic predisposes patients to problems with wound healing. Patients will often note that they develop "paper-thin" scars. Patients also have excessively flexible, loose joints. These 'hypermobile' joints can be easily and frequently dislocated. Finally, fragile blood vessels leave patients experiencing easy bruising, even an increased tendency to serious episodes of bleeding.

Often there are videos of people who are contortionists who can wrap their shoulders behind their back or pull the skin far from their face. These people likely have Ehlers-Danlos Syndrome. There are people who do not have the full blown disease and may express a variant. The reason this is important to a cosmetic result is their scars tend to stretch out and they are more likely to have loose skin. Additionally in a BBL their skin strength may be compromised and over time the butt may droop as a result of the weight of the butt.

An easy clinical diagnostic sign of potentially am EDS variant can be performed with these two tests. If you can touch the tip of your nose with your tongue you are among 10% of the general population. 50% of the people with EDS can do this (Gorlin's sign). Another test is by bending and touching your thumb to your forearm with is demonstrated by 20% of the population. Having both of these abilities may be a sign of the EDS variant. It is not necessarily a contraindication to surgery but the patient would be warned of the potential risks in the healing process.

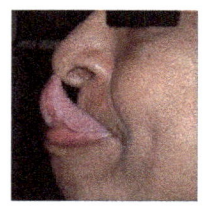

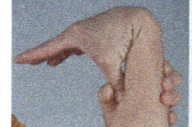

If you are interested in having your skin tighter after liposuction your options include:

1. **cutting and removing the skin**. No treatment has the potential to make you skin as tight as simply removing the loose skin surgically. Depending on where the skin is removed, that changes the name of the procedure.

BODY REGION	PROCEDURE NAME
on the abdomen	tummy tuck (abdominoplasty)
on the upper back	upper body lift (bra lift)
on the lower back	lower body lift
belly and lower back	circumferential body lift (total body lift)
on the arms	brachiopexy

on the neck	neck lift (submentoplasty)
inner thighs	inner thigh lift (medial thigh lift)
outer thigh	outer thigh lift (lateral thigh lift)

2. Skin tightening technologies all work on the same basic premise. Just as you heat a piece of chicken in a frying pan it shrinks, the concept is the same. Heating the collagen fibers causes skin contraction.

Collagen protein is a compound of 3 polypeptide chains, which are involved in a triple helix structure. The process of thermal contraction of collagen begins with denaturing the triple helix. The organized structure turns into a gel like structure. The collagen contraction occurs by the cumulative effect of the "unwinding" of the triple helix due to the destruction of the cross linking. The shape, the length and the diameter of the collagen fibers are changed as the reorganization of collagen takes place.

A. The heat can be applied <u>**under the surface of the skin.**</u> Such examples are:

a) radio frequency - a probe is placed under the skin that heats the collagen to 50-60°C (for example ThermiTight®)

b) laser- a laser probe is inserted under the skin and a laser fires to heat the tissue, there are many different lasers with various wavelengths (Smart lipo™, Lipotherme™)

c) j plasma (now called Renuvion®) - The **J-Plasma®** device starts with helium gas and uses radiofrequency (RF) energy to ionize it, turning it into cold helium **plasma**. This too heats the tissue and can cause contraction.

The nice thing about these technologies is that they are treating the intended target at the level of the target under the skin. In the author's opinion, the results from any of these technologies are not as good as the surgical procedures listed above. Speaking to many of my colleague with this equipment they agree.

The things that suck about these technologies from the doctors standpoint, they are expensive for us to buy. These toys can sometimes cost $80,000 to $200,000+. Then the disposable parts that have to be thrown out between patients can cost $300-$800 per case. Many machines also have a 'pay per click' functionality that costs the doctor more money to run the machine. Then there is maintenance to the device and warrantees, etc and owning these devices can be pricey for the doctor. Then in 2 years something new comes out that everyone is talking about and this becomes old technology.

This may stop a doctor from buying one. On the flip side, if a doctor owns one they may push this treatment on their patients to pay off the expense they just made on less than ideal candidates.

B. The heat can also be delivered **on top of the skin**, which intuitively the question becomes can the deep tissues become heated high enough to reach the needed temperature without burning the skin?

Bipolar, tripolar or multipolar electrodes are all different types that can deliver the heat needed for skin contraction. There are probably 100 machines that use different energy, all claiming to have the best penetrance4. (Ulthera®, Thermage®)

Infrared heat can also create heat on the skin and penetrate deep in the tissue (Skintyte™).

C. Burning the skin is another consideration but cannot be performed on darker skinned people and must be done very superficial. Skin on the body regenerates poor due to the lack of pilosebacious units compared to the face. These burns can take place with lasers or chemical peels. This is not a reliable technology for body skin tightening.

D. Micro needling is another alternative but is better for stretch marks than truly tightening skin.

E. Cold lasers I do not believe is truly effective (red and blue lights) for skin tightening.

In summary, surgery which removes skin is the most effective in treating loose skin especially for people with more than a pinch of skin. The options listed in choice "A" are ok but not as good as surgery. The options in "B" will make a very small difference, not as good as "1" or "A". The other options are not significant players in skin tightening.

If your doctor anticipates you have loose skin the things you can do are:

BEFORE SURGERY

Lose weight

Fat under the skin is like a hammock filled with rocks. If you take off all the rocks at once, the hammock doesn't have a chance to come up nicely and will spiral out of control. That is similar to what liposuction does to skin with poor elasticity. On the other hand, if you take off one rock at a time, the hammock has time to come back slowly in a controlled fashion. This is what happens with weight loss. When you loose 0.5 - 2 pounds per day the skin will retract more than removing all the fat in one shot. If you are getting lipo, losing weight may help your skin retract. However, loosing too much weight may result in not having enough fat for your butt. Again, a BMI of 24-28 is all you usually need for a 'natural full BBL".

AFTER SURGERY

1. Lymphatic massages will help the skin retract

2. Wearing the proper fitting garment. Too tight is not good!

3. And pulling the skin up in the garment. If you have a fold of skin that hangs over your underwear before surgery you are likely going to have it after. It can be worse when the fat is removed. On the next page is a woman who I feared it would be worse. She listened to my suggestion and her skin behaved much better than anticipated. The left is her before picture, the right her after.

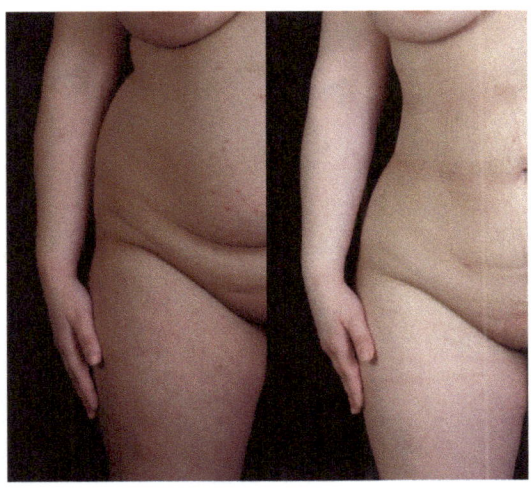

This is covered in other chapters but the fat is essentially the glue under the skin. If you pull the skin up in the faja especially in the first 10 days, and support it with foam or a board to keep it up, it can result in a more favorable result.

What does loose skin look like after lipo?
After liposuction if the skin does not retract well, you essentially wearing a suit that is too big for you. Imagine wearing a t shirt that it a few sizes too big. You cannot tuck it in, and you cannot trim it. You have to find a way to get the material to make contact with the skin. It will appear wavy on the surface. This is how the skin may sit. You may believe it is irregular lipo and your doctor did a crappy job

with lipo, but it may just be loose skin that has no where to sit.

The belly button hold up the middle of the belly skin and the skin may be lifted above it. This can create something that resembles a rainbow effect on the skin (see photo). Additionally zones of adhesion can be present on the lower abdomen and some people have them on other areas of the back or belly which creates fold.

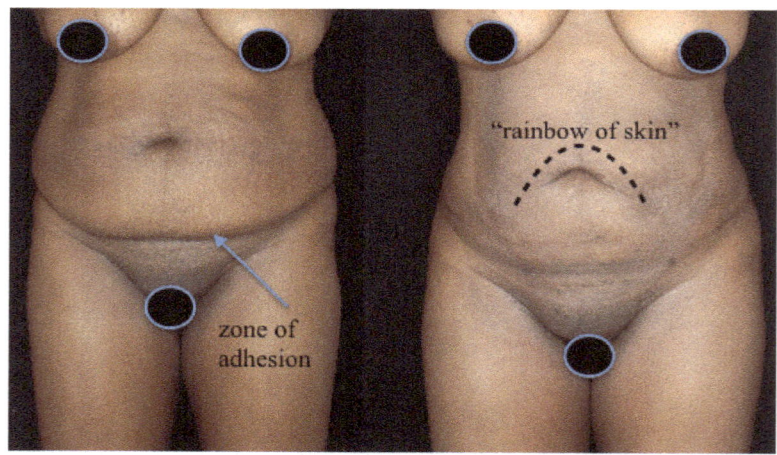

Before   After

Chapter 5: Cellulite and weird skin on the ass

"My bitch is bad and boujee I still treat her right, she gon hit up Dr. B got no cellulite."
                                                            Yuri Joness

Cellulite refers to the appearance of dimples or 'cottage cheese' in the skin of women which occurs most commonly on the thighs and butt. While many of these women are overweight and past puberty, it can be found in anyone. Multiple theories about why it happens exist, and can be quite upsetting to patients because of the uneven appearance.

Fun fact: Men do not get cellulite. The reason women get cellulite and men do not can be answered on a microscopic level. It is the pattern of their connective tissue under their skin. In women the pattern of collagen is in a **perpendicular orientation in women while in men it is in a** cross pattern.. When weight is gained in a woman the fat will deposit unevenly in these spaces between the collagen fibers and this pulls down on the skin unevenly. This gives an orange peel appearance to the skin. Because in men, the fat is buried in the more horizontally oriented collagen network we do not see the same effects on the external skin. Who runs the world? Yeah, still girls.

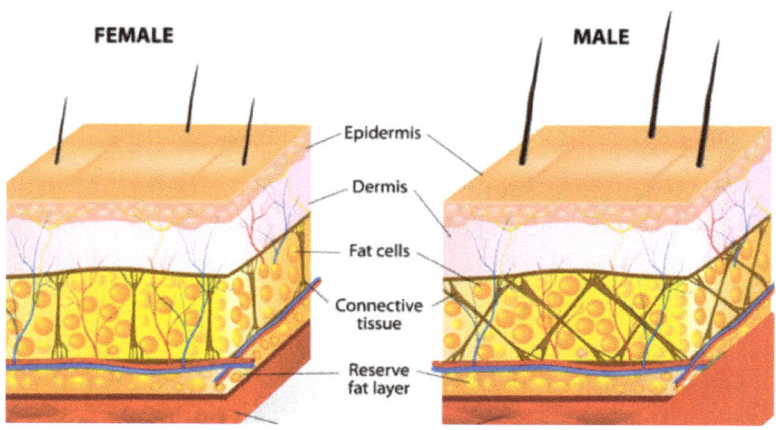

There are many procedures and creams that boast their ability to fix cellulite. Treating cellulite is the holy grail that there truly is not a great answer for. Most of the creams create a temporary tightness that hides the cellulite for a short amount of time. Many treatments and massages create swelling in the skin to again, camouflage the cellulite. When the swelling goes away, the cellulite is back starring you in the face.

Endermologie is FDA approved for the temporary improvement of cellulite as are products like VelaShape and Velasmooth. It creates swelling and temporary tightening through a combination of either infrared light, bipolar radiofrequency (RF) energy, massage, and gentle suction and hides the cellulite temporarily.

I am not a fan of Cellulaze™, which is essentially smart lipo for the superficial skin. I do not think it can safely do an adequate job breaking up cellulite in the superficial skin without damaging the skin.

Again, I'm not trying to be Debbie Downer, but it pisses me off seeing people taken advantage of. Is there anything that works? It depends on the severity and the degree of improvement that you are expecting.

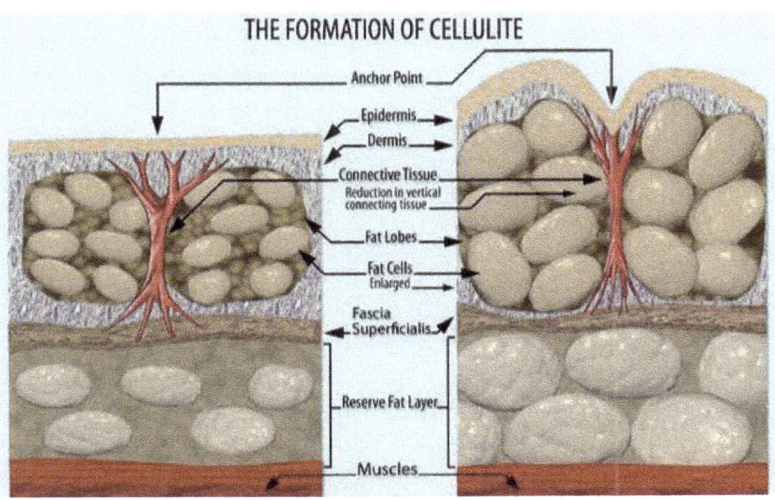

Looking again at the figure above, we see the formation of cellulite when there is a disproportionate amount of fat just under the skin, being tethered down by collagen fibers creating a dimple in the skin. Once you understand the reason it is there, it becomes easier to figure out if the advertised treatment will work. These are the things that can show some improvement to treat cellulite.
1. massive rapid weight loss- a large Scandinavian study showed a decrease in cellulite after rapid massive weigh loss.
2. Cellfina®- I was quite excited about this device when it came out because it makes sense to me. It breaks the fibers that create the dimpling and the fat is re-equilibrated to become smoother. How has it done? It

has a 72% 'it was with it' rating on the Real Self website as of today. In comparison to something like Botox, that has a 96% satisfaction rating. In the device's defense i do believe that it is operator dependent, not so much in doing the procedure (that seems easy), but in deciding if an area will respond well to a treatment and establishing expectations with a patient. It is not a cheap treatment, and it cannot be. The disposables alone are very expensive for a doctor to purchase for each treatment session. I still tell patients to look into this treatment if I believe they would benefit from it, even though I neither own the machine nor have any financial gain in referring it out.

3. Subcision - this is essentially doing the same thing as Cellfina® without the bells and whistles. it is breaking up the fibers that are tethering the skin down. When I do a BBL if a patient really doesn't like the cellulite they start out with, I will go in with a nokor needle (strong needle that is not hollow) or "pitch fork" to try to improve it a little. The same can be used for acne scars or any tethered down scar. I do not charge for this service, and I advise patients to expect a modest. Initially it will look like it is gone, because the patient is laying down on the table and the fat and skin is distributed differently. And for weeks it looks like it is gone because of the resultant swelling from the

procedure. When the swelling dissipates, it will likely return. Better, but it will likely still be there. If you are getting a BBL done just to improve cellulite, you are probably best spending your money elsewhere.

4. Adding filler into the depression of cellulite. It can be done with a filler depending on how deep and where the cellulite it. These are not without risk. General risks include, bruising, discomfort, infection just like any procedure. Products such as Sculptra® can cause granulomas, Radiesse® can cause skin necrosis or lumps if injected too superficially, as most fillers can.

Here's where I think a lot of doctors get into trouble. Hopefully you can learn this to make a good decision about your BBL.

Many people have loose skin on their lower back into their butt. it is commonly accepted that loose skin on the belly happens and is treated with a tummy tuck. For some reason, people have a hard time believing that there is loose skin that can form on the back. They are even more resistant to getting a scar on their back to treat it. I cannot explain this phenomenon.

Loose skin on the lower back can sabotage your hopes for a nice butt in a few ways. This is discussed fully in the chapters dedicated to weight loss and loose skin. This is how it can affect the appearance of cellulite on the butt.

The skin in the lower back and the butt cannot be supported in its proper position. When you lay down your butt will probably look smooth because the skin is laid out smoothly, like a pancake batter in a frying pan. When you stand up it becomes evident as the weight of the loose skin hangs and actually folds over the butt and the fibers tugging he skin inward creates a hooding over the tethered skin. This is because the skin envelope is larger than the surface area it needs to cover and the weight of the skin drips down the butt because of gravity. The skin is connected as it should be, by fibers that connect the skin to the deeper tissues.

When gravity is taken out of the equation it looks like the cross section of an orange.

Each little wedge in this slice is like a compartment separated by fibrous connective tissue, connecting the skin (rind) through the fat (juicy fruit part) to the muscle (center core).

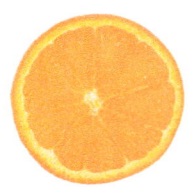

When you stand up, because the skin is pulling down and the uneven distribution of fat in the little sections is not full to capacity the orange slice will weep down. This can look like cellulite or indents where fat can simply be placed. If the actual REAL cause of the problem (loose skin) is not addressed, you will only be camouflaging the problem and it makes for a disappointing fix. Unless you only want to be seen in pants or laying on your belly.

Patients may think, who cares if I am just hiding a problem? Just add the fat. You can try to camouflage the problem by adding fat to these little compartments of irregularities, but here is the problem for the doctor (any doctor):

　　　　a. the surgery is done laying down and you can only see these things while standing
　　　　b. even if you remember where the defect is and mark them with a marker while standing, you won't know if you fixed them because, AGAIN, you are laying down when it is corrected
　　　　c. when you swell the problem looks likes its gone, when the swelling subsides, the problem comes back

Is it possible to fix with injections alone? Maybe. But it has little to do with skill, or artistry, it really is purely luck if it's fixed with fat addition of fat rather than subtraction of skin.
A better way to fix the problem is to actually make a cut

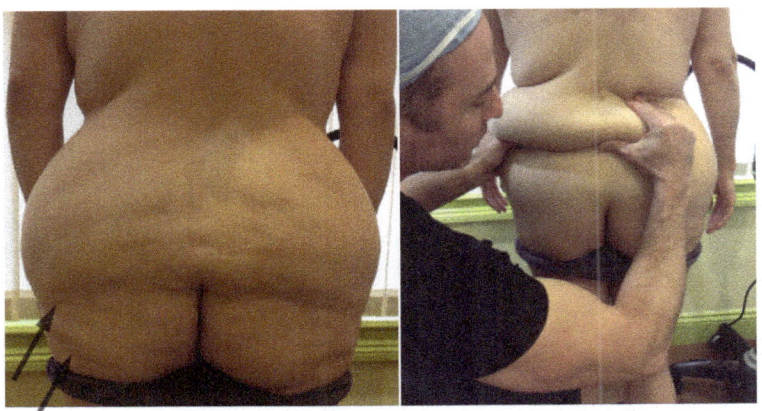

I like to demonstrate this with my consults. The butt on the left appears indented and not smooth as a result of loose skin. When it is repositioned in the proper place, true, the butt looks smaller, but it is smooth. This is now a good place to start adding fat. Adding fat to fill in the butt on the left will often leave a patient and a doctor frustrated and disappointed.

along the panty line and pull the skin up. This hoists the skin to the proper position and allows the extra skin to be removed. This addresses the problem head on instead of hiding the problem. I know it sounds crazy but this scar when it follows the shape of the butt and is put in the right spot can make the waist look totally snatched, lift the butt, and make the butt look fire! Take a look a these follow up pics of a patient who I did, just that!

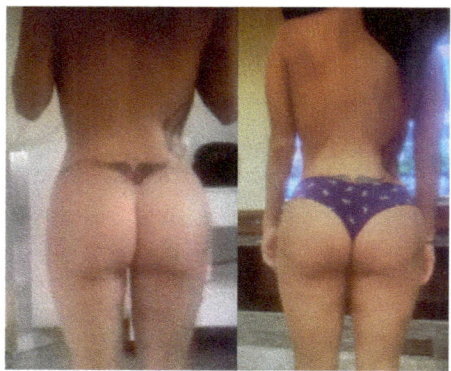

This is called a lower body lift when performed alone. If combined with a tummy tuck it is called a circumferential body lift or a belt lipectomy.

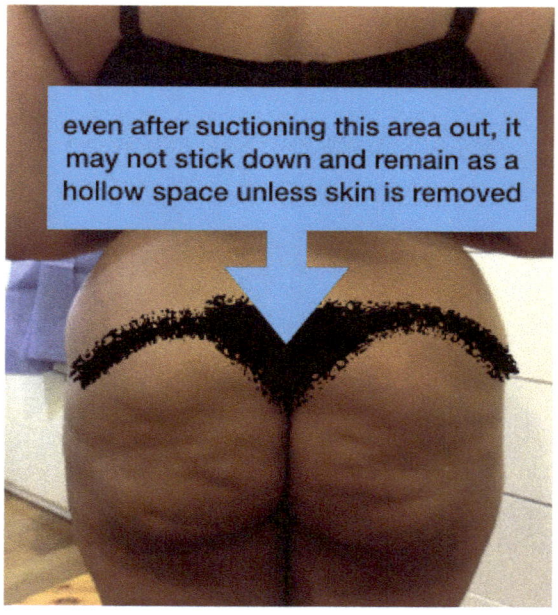

Chapter 6: BBL after massive weight loss

*"Sometimes I like slim, sometimes I like thick
Sometimes I combine them and I like them slick."*
                                                Fabolous

Much of this information overlaps with the chapter about loose lower back skin, but I want to make sure you don't miss this!

So you lost 100 pounds! That's incredible! Congratulations on your accomplishment! Maybe you are surprised to see a lot of loose skin everywhere? And where did that butt go??? I have treated many weight loss patients anywhere from 30 pounds to 200 pounds and these patients typically want all the extra skin gone to rock their new body. Unfortunately they will have to trade the skin for scars. Most do not mind.

These patients may need multiple surgeries with multiple phases including brachiopexy (arm tuck), abdominoplasty (tummy tuck), lower body lift, upper body lift, inner thigh lift, breast lift, or a neck lift to name a few. These surgeries are beyond the scope of this book so I will focus on what happens to the butt.

The butt is largely made up of fat and therefore melts away if you continuously loose weight. These patients, not as a fault of their own, run towards the finish line of a goal weight, with their bariatric surgeon, family, and friends pushing them along. While running, they are not looking or thinking of what's behind them (literally) to see what the effects on their butt are.

Some of the problems that occur after massive weight loss in the butt are:

1. A pure loss of volume. The butt is basically deflated.

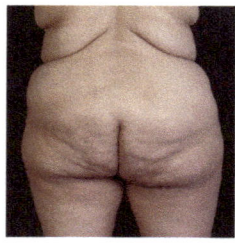
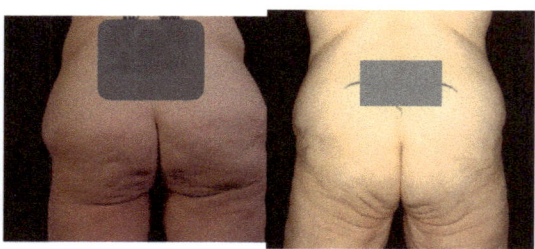

2. In addition to their loss of fat volume in their butt their lower back skin often drips into their upper butt. This gives the illusion that there is still some volume in their butt however it is just misplaced skin that is creeping beyond its turf. This can lead to a hump in the upper butt that looks like it is in need of simply filling the space below the hump up.

3. The other cosmetic deformity in the butt are these random pockets of cellulite which basically appear because the spaces between certain collagen fibers loose fat and the fibers still hold the skin in the original position so the skin weeps over them like a sad plant.

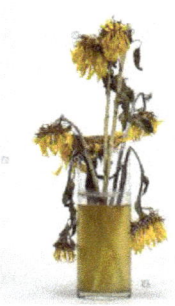

I like to demonstrate this by taking two pictures.

One standing up without any underwear.

A second picture holding the skin in the proper position. You can see all the irregularities improve and the skin hump disappear.

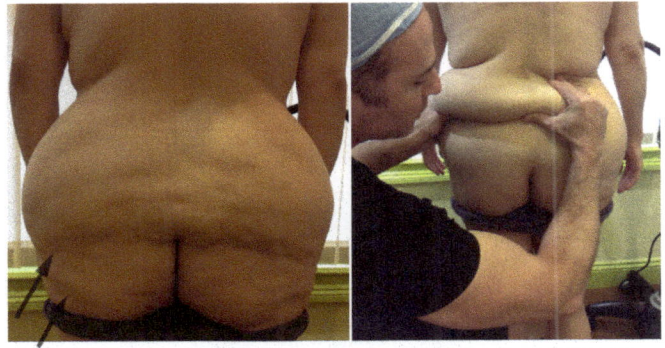

I like to demonstrate this with my consults. The butt on the left appears indented and not smooth as a result of loose skin. When it is repositioned in the proper place, true, the butt looks smaller, but it is smooth. This is now a good place to start adding fat. Adding fat to fill in the butt on the left will often leave a patient and a doctor frustrated and disappointed.

Now here are the problems with this patient:
1. They many times have to be ok with a scar that goes above the butt to remove the extra skin and put the butt in its true position. (This is a true butt lift btw) The butt will actually be in the right spot. This can make the butt appear actually smaller, but it will be smoother and if at the same time or in the future if you wanted to add fat the but would look much better.

SIDE VIEW

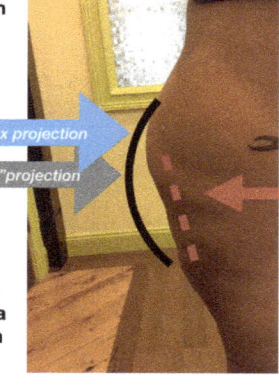

1. The loose skin from side view will make the maximum projection in the wrong position,

current max projection

based off this, "the wrong ideal max" projection

and it will be impossible to fill in the space to make a new max projection point.

2. It will make flat spots that cannot be popped out because the skin will hood here it no matter what will be attempted.

After lower body lift SIDE VIEW

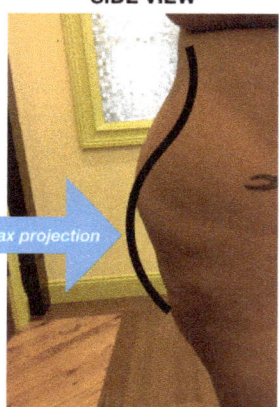

1. The loose skin removed will create a better upper butt curve allowing for the maximum projection to be in the correct place.

max projection

2. Flat areas are tented up allowing them to be filled and therefore rounded out, without loose skin hooding over it.

Personally, when done correctly the incision could like quite nice in the right spot and hidden under the underwear. Here is an example of someone who looked very well with a lower body incision that followed the arch of her butt.

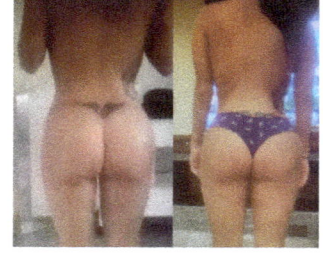

56

2. Trying to simply fill in the butt with fat is very difficult and unpredictable. Imagine the cross section of an orange. As we lose weight we loose fat in these sections of the fruit slice as well. However we do not lose it equally. We will loose no fat in some sections, 10 cc in one section, 5 cc is another, 2 cc in another etc. This causes some compartments of fat to collapse and weep down, and

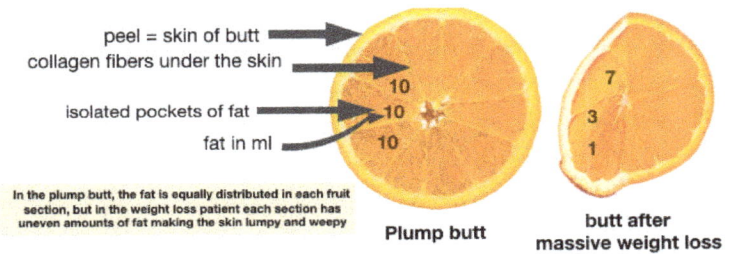

Plump butt — butt after massive weight loss

others will stand proud. When the patient stands up gravity pulls the tissue down and creates an uneven presentation on the skin.

When the patient lays down gravity is not pulling down and everything is spread out evenly and the defects are not appreciated.

So here are the problems trying to fix these spots by just injecting fat:

a. When you lay down (that is how the surgery is being performed) it is impossible to see the problem. We always mark the patient standing up. Most of the world sees us in this position (unless you are a porn star). We can mark the spots where the problems are and we can guess how much fat is needed in each spot to fill it up, but we cannot confirm we filled it up appropriately until months down the road at a follow up appointment. At this point, the swelling is gone, the fat that is going to take - took, and again the person is standing up. Is it possible to 'get it right' by just filling in the spots with fat? It would be like winning the lottery. It is not impossible but it would just be pure luck.

b. It is very difficult and again, basically absolute pure luck to push a 5 mm blunt tip cannula into a tiny pocket of

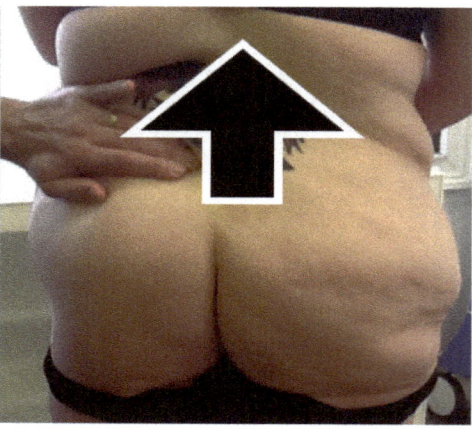

When the skin is repositioned up, the unequal distribution of fat is no longer noticed as the effects of gravity are removed and the skin is placed in the proper spot.

Note the smoother left side where the upward tension is being applied.

fat, confirm you are in, guess how much fat you need to put in to make it match the neighboring tissue, and make all of it live there without any of it going away. To use the orange analogy, that is asking the doctor to fill hundreds of these tiny fruit wedges equally by feel.

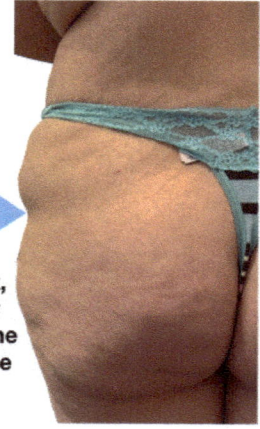 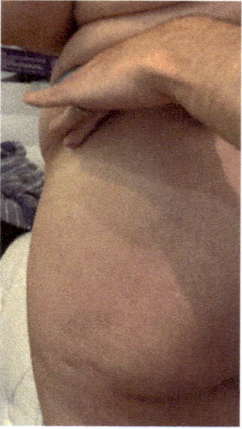

This depression is the symptom. The disease is the extra skin above the dip. To look its best, the loose skin above should be removed to allow for a smooth fill.

If you have Step throat, do you treat the runny nose? Or do you treat the bacteria that caused the illness?

You are much better pulling the skin up to create a tighter envelope and inject like a fresh virgin butt.

This is also true of the side of the hips. Particularly after massive loss or even lipo of the sides of the hips, these small sections of fat pockets are just too hard to individually fill. It is nearly impossible to get a satisfactory result without cutting the skin and making the areas tighter to fill them again.

3. These patients just dropped mad weight. Literally, a small person just came off their body. Along the journey they have been chasing the numbers on the scale. Skin has weight to it. The skin will not go away, so many patients believe they are still fat when they come to my office asking to get the BBL that they had been dreaming of. Unfortunately, without realizing it, they overshot their ideal weight for a BBL. The last thing these patients want to do is gain weight again. Trust me, I have asked, "how about gaining another 20 pounds?" and I had to be prepared to get wacked in the head. It is best to get the consultation for a BBL not before you hit what you perceive to be your ideal weight, but before it.

4. When you try to make an appointment for a consultation with a doctor many have a BMI restriction they follow. In the defense of the doctor, there are multiple studies showing those with a BMI of less than 32 have less complications with surgery, with anesthesia, an easier recovery, and a higher patient satisfaction. The massive weight loss patient can have a falsely high BMI. This may prevent the patient from getting an appointment to see the doctor, or even cause the patient to keep losing weight only to not have enough fat for the BBL procedure. Please check out the BMI (Chapter 7) for a more thorough discussion.

Many times the receptionist is given the BMI requirements, and he/she may deny a patient a consultation without knowing that they lost a massive amount of weight. Not a mistake of their own, perhaps the issue of BMI and weight loss was never discussed with the person answering the phone.

<u>Special</u> <u>cases</u>:
If the patient has extra skin in the butt and a limited fat supply and wants a 'shelf' on top of the butt one can make the same upper incision above the butt.

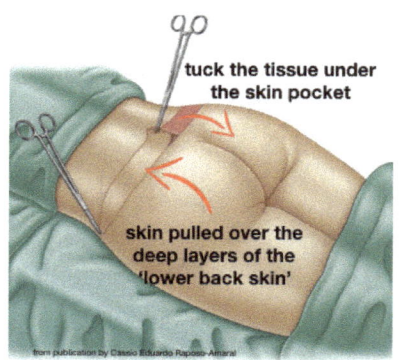

This is referred to as a dermal pedicle flap. In this situation the outer layer of skin is removed as shown and the deeper tissue (meat) is tucked under the skin. This can give fullness to the upper butt.

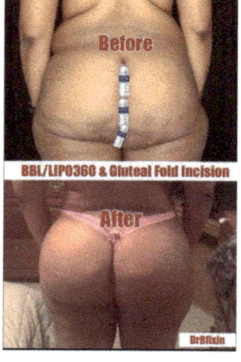

Another unique approach to patients with loose skin is an incision in the lower gluteal crease. This is good in a patient with very asymmetric folds (left) or someone who has little to no break from the butt to the leg and wants more of a pop (next page).

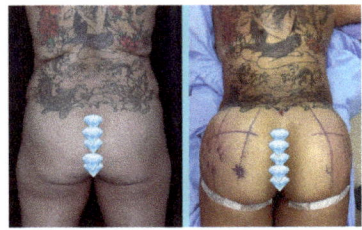

In Summary:

In an ideal world, the bariatric surgeon will prepare you before the weight loss journey of the outcome of loose skin and the potential desire to remove the loose skin. It is best to establish a relationship and a preliminary plan during the weight loss journey rather than at the end of the journey. It is best to do the BBL before the final weight goal has been achieved. To do the other potential skin removing procedures (basically anything requiring a real incision) it is best to hit the final goal weight and then be stable at that weight for at least 6 months or beyond.

Chapter 7: BMI (whats the deal?)

"Hold the weight, more to gain, more at stake. I got shit to do, had to move, with the crew away."
Travis Scott

What is BMI anyway?

BMI stands for body mass index. BMI is derived from a simple math formula. It was devised in the 1830s by Lambert Adolphe Jacques Quetelet, a Belgian astronomer, mathematician, statistician and sociologist. It is just two numbers: weight divided by height squared. BMI is an **inaccurate** measure of body fat content and does not take into account muscle mass, bone density, overall body composition, and racial and sex differences.

BMI can't distinguish between fat and muscle, which tends to be heavier and can tip more toned individuals into overweight status, even if their fat levels are low

If you want to know your BMI just google BMI calculator and plug in the numbers.

According to the CDC, here's what your number means:
- Below 18.5: underweight
- 18.5 to 24.9: normal
- 25 to 29.9: overweight
- 30 and over: obese

A 2016 study in the International Journal of Obesity looked at over 40,000 people across all population groups. They reported that more than 30% of people in the normal-BMI category are cardio-metabolically unhealthy based on their blood pressure readings and metabolic labs (such as "good" and "bad" cholesterol, triglycerides, glucose, and C-reactive protein). In addition, half of overweight people and 29% of obese people were healthy based on their health markers. The study estimated that as many as 74 million people who are considered to be unhealthy based on their BMI are, in fact, healthy.

Despite its limitations and infamous counter examples, why are we still using it?
1. BMI correctly categorizes people as having excess body fat more than 80 percent of the time.
2. No good other options exists right now

Other options have been proposed, such as:

Waist Circumference The National Heart, Lung, and Blood Institute recommends that your waist circumference be less than 40 inches for men, and less than 35 inches for women.

Waist-to-Height Ratio A waist-to-height ratio of more than 0.5 may put you at higher risk for heart disease and diabetes.

Waist-to-Hip Ratio The World Health Organization categorizes high risk as a ratio above 0.85 for women and more than 0.9 for men. You can calculate your waist-to-hip ratio by taking your waist circumference and dividing it into your hip circumference.

Body Fat Percentage You can measure this value with various methods, various methods, including skinfold, bioelectrical impedance (BIA), underwater weighing (hydrostatic), and dual energy X-ray absorptiometry (DXA). Skinfold and BIA values are easy to obtain but may be inaccurate. Meanwhile, hydrostatic and DXA are more accurate, but they can be costly, and the tools used to determine these values are less prevalent in clinical settings. MRI is another option but can be quite costly.

Despite these different approaches, experts agree that where you store your fat is most important. People who have extra weight in the abdominal area tend to be at the highest risk for disease because the fat may be encasing vital organs. This is referred to as visceral fat. Visceral fat increases the risk of cardiovascular disease, diabetes, and major organ disease.

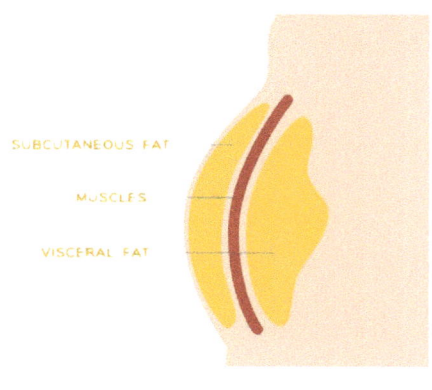

This is true of the surgical candidate. I have done consults on patients with a BMI of 26 but have a lot of visceral fat. Not only does visceral fat present a health risk to the patient but it will compromise your result for a procedure like a tummy tuck. That fat is under the muscle and around the organs and is not addressed with liposuction or a tummy tuck. Visceral fat will prevent my ability to make your stomach fat. So even though you are at a good number at 26 for surgery, it is not the best number for your particular surgical outcome.

On the flip side we have seen patients with a BMI of 34 with very little fat in their belly and back. They are looking for a BBL with lipo 360. We ask them to lose weight to get them to a BMI of 32. When they hit that number they have barely enough fat for the butt they desire.

We have seen this in the massive weight loss patient too. Their BMI may be 34 but it is because they are carrying so much extra skin and by them chasing a number on the scale, they literally melt away their butt. Their BMI with the extra loose skin will be erroneously high.

Other populations with problems with BMI being inaccurate include:

- **Asian People** Because Asians typically have relatively smaller bodies, a normal BMI is not a good measurement of these individuals' health risk. In other words, if you are Asian, your health risks may increase before your weight technically qualifies you as in the overweight category (BMI of 25 or higher).
- **Athletes** People who are extremely active have heavier bones and more lean muscle mass. This results in higher body weights and higher BMIs. However, lean muscle mass can actually increase metabolism, as well as improve conditions like heart disease and type 2 diabetes. Thus, an athlete with a high BMI may not necessarily be unhealthy.
- **Women Who Are Pregnant or Nursing** Women typically have a higher body weight and body fat percentage when nursing or pregnant, for the purpose of supplying nourishment to the baby (obviously not BBL candidates).
- **Nonpregnant Women** Compared with men, women generally have a higher percentage of body fat.
- **People Over Age 65** A BMI of less than 23 is associated with a higher health risk, and, according

to research, a BMI of 27 is the best in terms of mortality among this age group. Those with a higher BMI tend to carry more pounds of muscle compared with those with a lower BMI, which has a protective effect in terms of overall functionality, fall risk, and overall immunity.

I plugged my numbers into the BMI calculator. I am 6 feet tall and weigh 189 pounds. My BMI is 25.6. This classifies me as overweight. I am in excellent shape and clearly fit in the category of athlete, not to mention I carry an unusually large package between my legs (I wish, but its not too bad fyi).

In summary, BMI is not perfect. It is best for us as doctors to look at the whole picture.

As a patient, it may be frustrating when you want an appointment and the receptionist tells you that you cannot see the doctor because your BMI is too high. Even more frustrating, is loosing the weight to fit the BMI requirement for the office you wish to go to and being told that you don't have enough fat for the procedure and you need to gain weight again.

In my office I have a soft requirement for a BMI of 32. When I see you for a consult, I can better estimate and will tell you if you need to gain or lose weight before surgery. We tailor the goal weight to your presentation, health, and desires.

Chapter 8: Multiple surgeries at the same time?

"I really don't think I need buns of steel. I'd be happy with buns of cinnamon."
Ellen DeGeneres

A Brazilian Butt Lift typically consists of lipo 360. This refers to liposuction of the belly, back, and sides. Many patients chose to add other procedures at the same time. There are advantages and disadvantages to doing more surgery at the same time.

Advantages:
- **It can be cheaper.** It is often less expensive to do the second or third procedure at the same time. In my office, my anesthesia provider charges me by the hour. The first hour is most expensive and it decreases after the first hour. For that reason the additional surgery costs me less to perform it. We extend that discount to the patient, many doctors do likewise.
- **Recovery time is tough to come by.** For many people, it is difficult to take multiple long periods of time away from work. The average time off from a typical desk job is 10 days to 2 weeks. Adding another procedure at the same time usually does not extend the amount of days required off for recovery.

Disadvantages:
- It is a more difficult recovery
    - Sleeping can be difficult. After a tummy tuck you cannot sleep flat or on your belly. After a BBL you cannot sleep on your butt. This leads to people sleeping on your side or within a device (like an inner tube from a swimming pool) and some collateral pressure can inadvertently be placed on the butt.
- More anesthesia time, more risk
- Can compromise the result, more specifically the butt result
- If a tummy tuck is being performed at the same lipo as a fat transfer, the doctor may have to be more conservative with the liposuction to maintain the health of the tummy tuck flap
- Adding arms can make things more difficult to move around as people tend to depend on their arms to get up and hold themselves up more when they can't get up as well.
- The ideal BMI (body mass index - *check out the previous chapter*) for a tummy tuck is as low as you can be. The ideal BMI for a butt can be 27. If you show up to surgery in ideal tummy tuck weight, you may be too thin to have enough fat for a BBL. If you gain lots of weight for a BBL, you can jeopardize your tummy tuck result. Super aggressive liposuction during a tummy tuck is a bad idea and if too much visceral fat is gained, the skin will not be able to be pulled down as tight. '

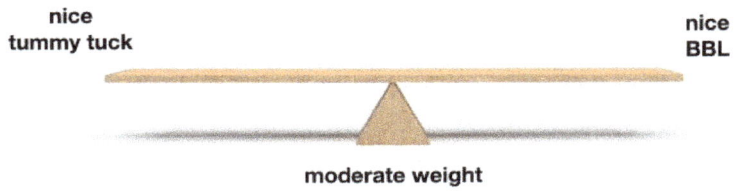

A BBL can be added on to almost any other type of cosmetic surgery case in my opinion except a rhinoplasty, eyelid or facelift surgery. The recovery period for a BBL

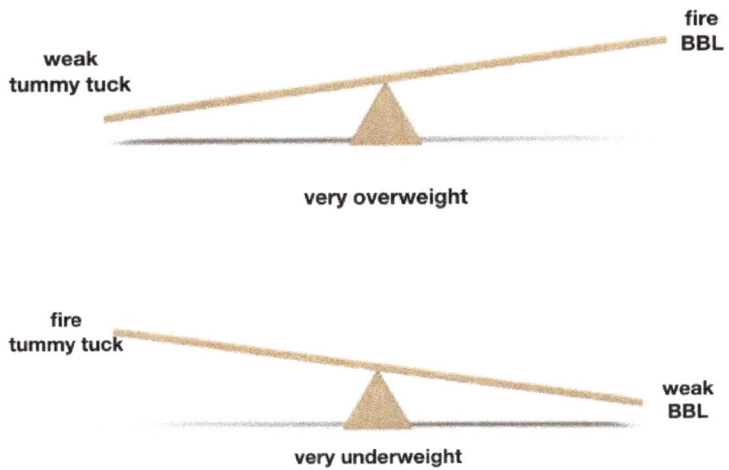

requires much of the time to be face down, especially while sleeping. This leads to a tremendous amount of gravity dependent swelling that manifests itself in the face. For eyelids it could cause extreme prolonged swelling and in an even worse scenario bleeding behind the eye that could even lead to blindness. For a facelift, excessive pressure on the face can lead to a collection of blood under the flap known as a hematoma that can cause the facelift flap to die off (necrosis). A rhinoplasty can also result in prolonged swelling of the nose that will usually sit in the tip of the nose and can stay there for an extended time. More importantly, if the bones are broken which oftentimes is the case during a rhinoplasty, the bones can shift if pressure if placed on the nose while sleeping on your belly.

For those considering butt implants, or even breast implants, the chance of infection must be taken very seriously. The treatment for such an infection can be devastating and is best avoided. A normal wound needs a bacterial load of 1,000,000 bacteria to get an infection. On an implant, that number is only 10,000 bacteria. Making an incision in a distant area with a large bacterial load can potentially compromise the implant and create an infection. The bacteria can enter the incision, travel in the bloodstream and seed on the implant. These dirty areas include, the mouth, nose, vagina, and perianal areas. It is for this reason I will never consider placing an implant at the same time of a rhinoplasty, inner thigh lift, or vaginoplasty. Many doctors do, it is my philosophy not to. I would even consider taking preventive antibiotics after implant surgery for a few months after an implant surgery if getting a surgery in one of the aforementioned areas.

It is well established in the cardiac literature that a heart valve requires premedication before surgical procedures. In the orthopedic literature after a total joint replacement it is recommended to take antibiotics before a surgical procedure for 2 years window after surgery. There are no such recommendations for cosmetic surgery implants. In 2010 I decided to take on the initiative to establish such guidelines. I spent a few weeks working on this but then got too busy and never finished. I do believe the need for such guidelines is there but I'm too busy making fat asses to finish it.

It is my belief, that going to the dentist for a cleaning, have periodontal or oral surgery one should take prophylactic antibiotics before surgery after any body implant. The most common antibiotics being Amoxicillin or Clindamycin (if penicillin allergic). There are published cases of people growing bacteria in cultures taken from around a breast implant that originated in the mouth. This was found in people who had a breast augmentation and a few weeks later had some periodontal surgery done.

In summary, there are some surgeries that are combined well together and others that are not. If you are healthy enough for a prolonged time under anesthesia, and your hemoglobin levels are solid enough to handle an expected drop after surgery, this can be a consideration to discuss with your doctor. As a consumer (patient) you should also consider potential fatigue of your surgeon. I have had patients come to me to fix problems they have acquired from other doctors, who in my opinion were careless. Most likely mistakes made by fatigue and too much in one surgery. We are human. Make sure your doctor isn't running a mill, and make sure he/she looks like they (the doctor) will survive 2-3 hours of lipo- it is a real cardio workout.

Chapter 9: Choosing your doctor

"Certified everywhere, ain't gotta print my resume."
Migos

Stay Woke!

This is going to piss off a bunch of people, but I don't really give a shit. I write this wholeheartedly for you, the patient.

This may go against many of the stuff you hear or read, but this is the truth. There is no substitute for experience. To make a blanket statement like, "make sure you go to a board certified plastic surgeon for this procedure" means nothing more than that person graduated medical school, did a residency in plastic surgery, and passed a written and oral exam. Yes, this is a great accomplishment but this means nothing about the experience this doctor has in this procedure, ethics, his or her artistic vision, skill of one's hands, compassion towards his or her patients, or ability to communicate. This procedure has gained the most popularity recently, and I am willing to hazard a guess that the people giving you this generalized advice has done probably less than a handful, and maybe even 0 BBLs during their residency training. There are many deaths associated with this procedure. Many of which are board certified plastic surgeons. There is nothing showing board certified plastic surgeons are less likely to cause a BBL death. Nothing.

This is a very politically charged issue, and tackling this issue is not the intention of this chapter. The only point is, I have met many Board certified plastic surgeons. Many are amazing doctors and they perform miracles daily. Many are my friends. Many are not. Not all of them perform cosmetic surgery. The requirements to graduate from a plastic surgery program for cosmetic surgery are minimal, and there is a possibility that the board certified plastic surgeon you are consulting with has never even done a Brazilian Butt Lift.

The American Board of Cosmetic Surgery accredits surgeons from various specialties after extensive additional training or experience in cosmetic surgery. To qualify to be board certified in Cosmetic surgery, one must be board certified in their primary specialty, have completed a credentialed cosmetic surgery training program (dedicated to cosmetic surgery) or prior to 2013 have performed over 1500 cosmetic cases (this experience route is no longer an option). After that, the surgeon must take a written and oral exam, maintain CE credits, and recertify after a certain amount of years. Even *these* doctors may do very minimal Brazilian Butt Lifts.

To simply call yourself a cosmetic surgeon says nothing about your experience or training. There are doctors who call themselves cosmetic surgeons with a vast amount of experience, and some with little to none.

So there are three groups of surgeons I am talking about here:

1. Board Certified Plastic Surgeons,
2. Board Certified Cosmetic Surgeons, and
3. Cosmetic Surgeons (not board certified)

When Plastic Surgeons bad mouth other specialties they often use broad strokes and describe someone who took a course and calls themselves a cosmetic surgeon. This is misleading to put this person in the same category as a board certified cosmetic surgeon. It is a pet peeve of mine when someone asks a question on a site like Real Self and the question is insufficiently addressed, but instead a plug is made for "make sure you seek care from a board certified plastic surgeon". Almost as though they are programmed to write the same script for every question. There are great board certified plastic surgeons and there are great board certified cosmetic surgeons. There are horrible board certified plastic surgeons and there are horrible board certified cosmetic surgeons. Just there are great plumbers and horrible plumbers, great cops and horrible cops, etc. Getting through a program, answering questions correctly on a test, says very little about many other important qualities when choosing a doctor.

For more information about the difference between plastic and cosmetic surgery please see https://www.americanboardcosmeticsurgery.org/

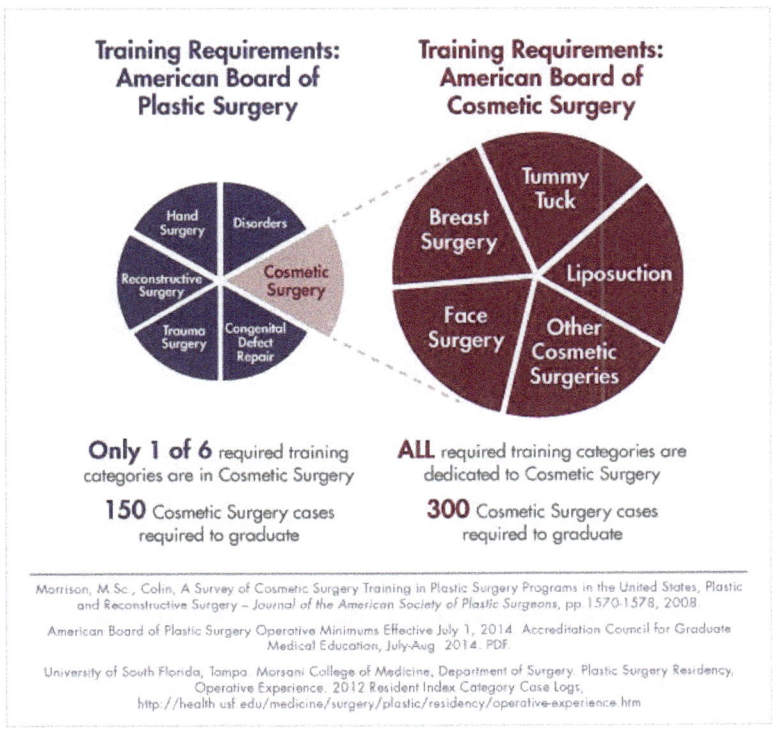

The point is this. In the book Talent is Overrated: What Really Separates World-Class Performers from Everybody Else by Geoff Colvin, the author explains that experience is king. He describes 10,000 hours of training will allow anyone to master almost anything, talent aside. In my opinion I do agree with this to a point. The Brazilian Butt Lift is not just about moving fat from point A to point B it is about much more than that.

I would look for a doctor who is well trained, and experienced but also understands the culture, and knows what a sexy woman should look like. Someone who looks like they would appreciate a nice butt in yoga pants. I would want my doctor to not only be an artist but a consumer. It should be someone you should feel comfortable talking to. Someone who you can share your desires to and not be embarrassed, and believe the doctor 'gets it'.

Someone who is approachable and who takes pride in their work. Someone who doesn't treat you like a pay check and done. See about the author for more details, just kidding (not really kidding though, fr).

My belief is any surgeon who has enough experience in the procedure and performs it in an ethical and safe way is qualified to do this surgery. It doesn't matter your surgical specialty as long as you have proper training in this specific surgery. Another belief is anyone performing any surgery should be trained in how to handle any complications that could be encountered. I have met surgeons who have performed surgery and failed to identify a problem after surgery, and others who had no idea on how to manage it and referred the patient elsewhere. If you have no idea on how to manage the complications inherent with the surgery, you should not be performing the surgery.

Now to do it well, that is another animal.

This procedure has a tremendous artistic demand. Imagine if we had 100 biologically identical woman. We would then assign 100 different well qualified surgeons do breast augmentations on each woman. If we lined up each woman and looked at their breast augmentation results it would be hard to distinguish which surgeon did what. Every person would look pretty similar.

I submit to you the same scenario with rhinoplasty (nose jobs). In this situation people would look quite different. Some could potentially look very bad. In my opinion, amount of skill required to do a rhinoplasty is much greater than that of a breast augmentation. A more seasoned surgeon in this situation would have a better result. The nose is to the face as the butt is to the body.

The Brazilian Butt Lift is a surgery that requires much skill, experience, know how, artistic eye, a shared vision between patient and doctor, and an understanding of cultural and urban trends, and did i say experience? Yes, a lot of experience. Not only for a great result but for a safe one.

Chapter 10: Price

"How much a dollar really cost?
The question is detrimental, paralyzin' my thoughts."
                              Kendrick Lamar

This chapter is to alert you how some clinics may be misleading and disingenuous and to make sure you know what you are getting.

A BBL {(Brazilian bull lift) usually encompasses liposuction 360. Liposuction 360 is liposuction of the entire belly, back and the sides. You should make that clear with the doctor you are going to see. You can get fat from the arms or legs and add that to the butt but these additional areas are usually additional guap $$$.

There is no standardized prices for lipo 360 BBL and is largely dependent on the doctor, region in the country, and what is included. The highest price isn't always the best, and the lowest price isn't always the worst. There are some real expenses that a doctor must absorb so I would be suspicious if the price is ridiculously low.

The range in the on realself.com they list the range of a BBL to be
 $2,400 - $10,500 with the average price of 6,525. On the website https://www.brazilianbuttlift.com/costs.html the range of cost is demonstrated to be between $2000 and $12,000, with an average cost of around $6,500. I do believe these numbers are a bit dated, and I am unsure when they have been published. The prices I have heard from my colleagues are on the average $11,000 upward to $20,000 plus in NYC and Beverly Hills. As of 2020, the fees

I charge in my office for lipo 360 and BBL is $12,499 which I believe is on the right side of the bell curve.

My BBL surgery consists of ultrasound assisted fat placement (which is extra equipment and time), we are accredited by the Joint Commission (the highest standard of facility excellence), we have a cell saver to recycle your lost blood, and we use general anesthesia with multiple board certified staff and top of the line ICU recovery room nurses. Care like this costs money and I would never want to cut any corners to jeopardize a patient's care. If I would have surgery in my office, I know I am in the safest place. If I did the surgery in a closet with a medical assistant, awake, I could do it for a lot less and make more money but this is not how I would treat my family or my patients.

These are some of the things that you should find out if they are included in the fee:

1. Does lipo include the stomach, back, and sides?

2. Does is include anesthesia, or is there a separate fee?

3. Are you getting general anesthesia?
    There are some doctors who do this awake with local anesthesia

4. Is a practitioner doing my anesthesia or is it done by the surgeon at the same time as my procedure?

5. Is there a separate facility fee?
    Some places charge a facility fee (commonly in hospitals) which can be $60/minute. This covers the staff in the operating room, and disposables gowns, drapes, tubing, blades, sutures, cannulas, containers, medications

and many other items that you do not need to know about. The question is however, is it already in the price?

6. Does it include the post operative garment or faja?

7. If I need a touch up is there an additional fee for this?

8. Are there any other expenses that I may incur aside from the amount listed on this proposal?

9. Is there a discount if I pay in cash?

10. Are there financing available? It is the same price if I finance?

Aside from the cost of surgery, there are other expenses you will likely be responsible for that are not part of the surgery. This should be kept in mind when you are getting your finances in order.

Remember to set aside money for:
1. medications
2. post operative massages
3. medical clearance and or blood work
4. travel and lodging if applicable
5. food
6. post operative garments

To pay for your surgery, the traditional methods of cash or credit will certainly apply everywhere. Some offices do offer a discount if paid in cash. You can certainly get a loan from friend, or family member, bank or your local credit union. Patients have borrowed from their 401k. Some offices finance surgery though their office but this becoming more rare. More commonly, most offices offer 3rd party financing. There are many such companies and it is best to find out which company the office you plan on having surgery works with, rather than the other way around.

Like most loans, your credit score is checked. Those with good credit have an easier time acquiring the loan with better rates. If you do get approved or have a card already (perhaps from even dental care you are getting), you can call up to add more money onto the credit limit. You can have someone else apply for a card with their permission and forms of their identification.

The more popular companies are listed here:

1. Care Credit - https://www.carecredit.com/
By far the most popular financing for your medical care. You can apply online in just a few minutes on your own, or with the help of the office. There is an interest free option of 12 months interest free. You generally start making the payments in monthly increments after the surgery.
The better credit you have, the more financing you qualify for and the more competitive interest rate, if you chose longer terms with interest.

Be good about your payments! If you are late for a payment, care credit will charge your interest for the entire amount from the beginning. We have seen a few patients go through this and the unexpected cost sucks.

2. Green Sky - Very similar to care credit however in our experience they are a little more forgiving than care credit with your credit score. Additionally, there is no penalty to pay it off early. So if you find a sugar daddy, have him pay it off ASAP; then cut him off.

3. Wells Fargo Health Advantage®

The Wells Fargo Health Advantage® card is worth a look if you've already got a credit card or loan through Wells Fargo.

4. Alphaeon Healthcare https://d.comenity.net/alphaeoncosmetic/

5. Parasail https://www.parasail.com/how-it-works/

6. Prosper Health https://www.prosper.com/

Chapter 11: Do you get what you pay for?

"In this country, you gotta make the money first. Then when you get the money, you get the power. Then when you get the power, then you get the women."

Tony Montana

You get what you pay for.

This expression along with, "if it sounds too good to be true, it probably is too good to be true," often holds true in life. We all want a good deal in most things we purchase and for something like a name brand television in a closed box, you can't really get it wrong.

You want the Sony 85 inch LED 4k television. You can look at Best Buy, PC Richards, Costco, Amazon, and various online stores. You know exactly what you are getting. You are getting a new Sony 85 inch LED 4k television, most likely with a warranty. This same tv you can buy at any of these stores will work the same.

Now let us consider your healthcare. For elective surgery, the patient has the luxury of looking to seek any doctor they want. Not all patients are looking for the best doctor or the most caring doctor some just look for the cheapest.

When doctors compete on prices it is a scary race to the bottom. The scariest part is someone will win.

There are costs to running business. The overhead for surgery is very high. My friend owns a surgicenter in NJ. He has podiatrists do bunioneictomies there.
The surgeon gets $3,000-$5,000 for the surgery.
The facility gets $30,000 from the insurance company.

💰 Anesthesia costs money
    -pay the anesthesia provider
    -well trained staff cost money
    -using disposable one time use instruments are expensive
    -malpractice for anesthesiologist
    -medications can be expensive
    -tubing and catheters are expensive
    maintaining all sterilizing equipment, surgical machinery is expensive
    -maintaining anesthesia machine every 6 months is expensive

💰 To have and replenish all the needed emergency medications in the office is very expensive

💰 To be an accredited surgical center and maintain certification and continued training is expensive

💰 All of the certifications to be in compliance with the Department of Health and the state is expensive.

💰 A surgeons malpractice insurance depending on their state can be between $50-$200,000 per year.

💰 Paying staff for preparing/booking/following up after surgery costs money

💰 Office costs

There is no way your surgery can be stupid cheap without cutting costs somewhere. I am not suggesting your doc is reusing disposable equipment (although I have heard of this). Even if your doctor is the nicest person on planet earth, he/she ain't building you an ass out of the kindness of his/her heart.

Recently a spa in New Mexico was shut down after spreading HIV doing vampire facials with a micro needling device without using the proper device. When you pay for cheap, sometimes you get cheap.

Find the most expensive, find the cheapest and find the doctor somewhere in between the two that you have a good feeling about. Don't look for the cheapest, because you will find the cheapest.

Chapter 12: It's cheaper in other countries

"My bi#ch, she Dominican Republic, but I'm Haitian, I ain't quit shufflin' in my feet, now I'm patient."
                                                    Kodack Black

It's cheaper in other countries. Yeah, it probably is.

There is a reason the United States has the best health care in the world. We have highly trained doctors, the highest of standards in our equipment, supplies, and materials used. We have standards put into place that can quite expensive for a private physician to abide by, but they are there to provide the safest environments for patients.

There are very talented doctors in other countries and there are man bad ones. These are my some of my concerns about having a patient fly to another country outside the US for surgery.

1. Standards of care
The United States Department of Health and Human Services' Centers for Disease Control and Prevention (CDC) warns that the quality of health care in overseas facilities may not be on par with the United States, and that foreign facilities are not always subject to the same health standards and regulations. Few overseas health facilities are accredited by the Joint Commission International (JCI), an organization that accredits overseas hospitals according to quality and safety standards similar to those in the United States.

There are some places that you do not meet your doctor until the day of surgery, Perhaps you do not even speak the language of the people caring for you.

2. Infection

The largest percentage (31%) of complications from surgeries overseas was infections. Many countries have infectious diseases such as; influenza, tuberculosis and some transmitted by mosquitoes that Americans and Europeans would not have built up a natural immunity against. We know too well the power of foreign viruses.

3. Other common surgical complications needed intervention

Other common complications reported by patients were dehiscence (where the wound opens up), contour abnormality, and hematoma (collections of blood in the site). These issues can happen or appear at any point during the healing process; not just immediately after surgery. You may have left the country your doctor is in and now cannot find a treating surgeon.

4. I have a post operative surgical problem, now what?

Personal medical insurance most likely will not cover a patient while out of the country, if a medical complication should arise, additional costs could be out of pocket. "Medical tourism" is typically excluded from travel insurance coverage.

If a complication arises at home there will be a need to find a local doctor willing to take on a case with complications which can be very expensive, not mention many doctors do not have malpractice insurance that would cover them for taking on such a case. Their other option is to travel back to the foreign country, which is not a great idea especially when not feeling well.

Additionally, there are no repercussions you can take to protect yourself versus wrongdoing. Meaning, you cannot sue a doctor from overseas.

I have seen patients that were told they got a small saline implant and instead got a large silicone implant.

We have seen a woman who went to Dominican Republic for a tummy tuck, and when she returned she wasn't feeling well so she went to the emergency room in NY. She discovered that in addition to her tummy tuck she had her kidney removed and apparently sold on the black market.

We have all heard of at least a few patients who went to another country for surgery and who do not return alive. There are such stories each month, they are a 'google' session away.

5. Checks and balances
The standards of care in the US are much greater than other countries. Medical errors can happen overseas or even in the US. The fact that the local physician out of the country may be unfamiliar with your case may pose additional challenges.

There are regulations that are in place for patient safety, such as the amount of liposuction that can be performed in one day. There are patients who actually want to have surgery in other countries to avoid these restrictions. These restrictions are in place not to limit how good you can look, they are there to protect you. There are parts of surgery that has been proven dangerous and the US has put restrictions and oversight in place to maintain your safety.

6. FDA regulations and standards

Sometimes inferior medical devices can be used such as breast implants for popular surgeries as breast augmentation. This would not be the case in the United States where implants are closely monitored by the FDA. Even the sterilization of instruments and sterile technique in the operating room is governed in the US by various agencies. These agencies do not govern in these foreign countries.

7. Traveling after surgery

One of the most popular cosmetic procedures today is the "Mommy Makeover", a combination of a tummy tuck with breast surgery. It is a long procedure and follow up care is very important. In most cases drains are used for 7 to 10 days. The patient must avoid strenuous activity, lifting and bending, making traveling through an airport with luggage difficult.

Preventing blood clots the day of surgery and throughout the recovery period is of extreme importance, and if missed can be potentially lethal. After any surgery you are at an increased risk of blood clotting in your legs, known as a DVT (deep vein thrombosis). Traveling on an airplane immediately after surgery greatly increases this risk due to the many hours of immobility.

The chance of acquiring an airborne infection on a plane after the stress of surgery is higher than staying local to your surgery facility.

8. Recovery

Recovering on a tropical beach is not a good option; the patient needs to stay out of the sun and out of the water is necessary to avoid scarring and infection. Being close to home with the support of family or friends is optimal.

Having your surgeon nearby is the safest situation. Enjoying a trip to a far off destination after healing is the best plan.

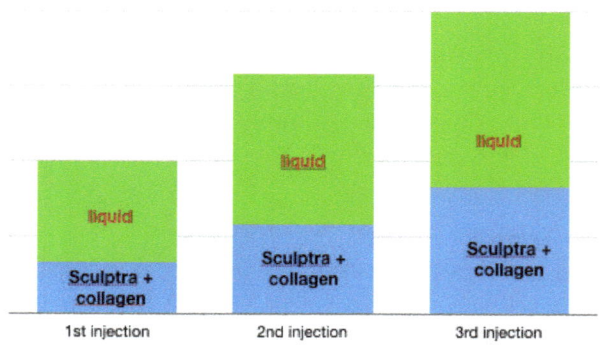

9. *Why* is the surgery cheaper?
There are excellent surgeons all over the world but many are able to have lower fees because they do not provide protection for patients such as medical malpractice or hospitals do not have liability insurance. Additionally, medical supplies, drugs, sutures, and implants are more expensive in the US with the added costs of FDA regulations

10. *Is* the surgery actually cheaper?
Estimated price for a simple tummy tuck
Flights $1,000/person x 2 $1000-2000
Hotel $800 for 1 week $800
3 Meals x 7 days $500
Surgery cost $3000-6000

Total $6300-9300

We all know someone who had a surgery overseas and looks great, and had a great experience. For every patient like this, we have heard the opposite story- a tragedy.

With every surgery there are risks. I do believe not as a responsible human, a friend, a father, or a brother your life is **not worth the gamble**. The risks of surgery are not just a tag line on a piece of paper, they are real. I do believe you are more at risk doing this traveling outside the US. The skeptics may see this as a doctor who wants your business and trying to get you to stay. I assure you I am doing well and don't need to convince anyone to get more business (that wasn't intended to sound cocky, sorry, just honest). I am not trying to compete with these clinics overseas. I truly believe you are putting yourself at a greater risk of injury, complications, and death. You are not ordering a pair of shoes from another country, you are putting your life in jeopardy. If you don't want to think of yourself, think of those around you who count on you.

As of July 2019, because of the growing number of deaths from cosmetic surgery, specifically in the Dominican Republic, new rules have been instituted a safer surgery for this going to DR. This is a step in the right direction for safety, but if these rules are enforced by the practitioner much of what the patient may have perceived as advantages of surgery abroad is negated.

Some of these guidelines for example include:
- patients must stay in the country at least 48 hours before surgery if the flight is less than 2 hours, or 5 days before if the flight is more than 2 hours.
- patients must stay in the country for 10 days for continental flights or 21 days for international flights.
- maximum of 5 liters of fat for lipo and if additional procedures, the maximum allowed is 3 liters.

- not more than 2 procedures at a time

I have heard from patients contemplating a trip to DR for their surgery stating,
"They can take out more than 5 liters of fat" - *this is no longer the case*
"I can have all the surgeries done at one time" - *this is no longer the case*
"It's mad cheap" - *if you add up travel and extended stay, the price is now much higher than it once was.*

These rules are good and are in place for your safety. Even with these rules I personally still see going to DR for surgery as a risk not worth taking.

Chapter 12: Alternatives to fat

"Them ass shots, them ain't real curves,"
Yo Gotti

I am not throwing shade on anyone trying to hustle to make some money, but f'ing people over really pisses me off. Maybe because I have been burned over the years because you trust someone and they f you. I am trying to write this as politically correct as possible but I so not taking advantage of people or seeing it done. That being said, lets get into it with an open mind....

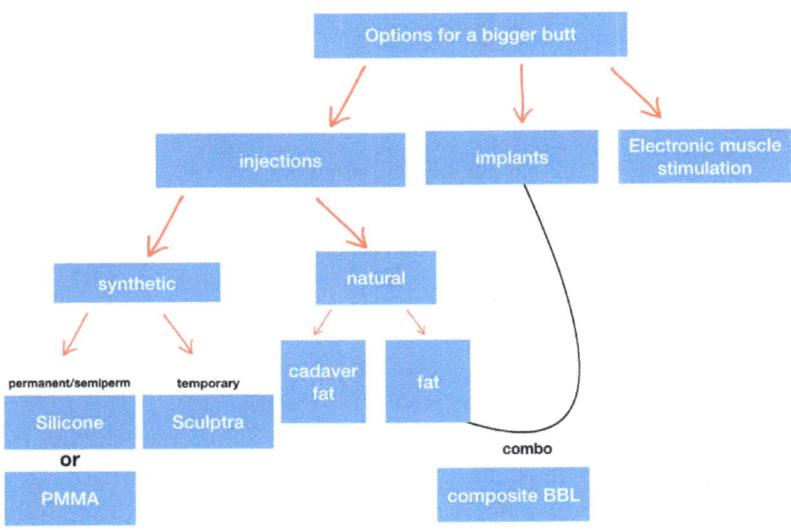

The gold standard for adding volume to the butt is fat. It is what G-d intended to be there and that is certainly the best option. But are there other options

If you are skinny and want to gain weight for the surgery that would be the best option. Check out Chapter 3 for information on that.

Silicone **implants** are an option but not my particular favorite option for large volume, particularly as the main component for volume. Using an implant with fat in my opinion makes for a better result than an implant alone. Check out Chapter 13 to read about that. Silicone injections should never be done in the butt (Chapter 14).

Now that we got that out of the way, lets go over fat alternatives. There is really no cost effective alternative to fat but a popular alternative is:

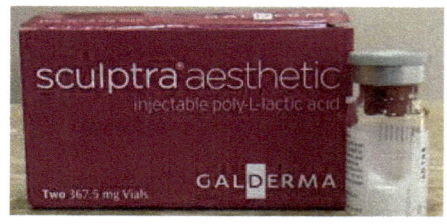

Sculptra®, or poly-l-lactic acid (PLLA), is a dermal filler used for skin and soft tissue augmentation and only FDA approved for the face. It is appropriate to inject in the butt as long as the patient is aware it is off label. PLLA stimulates the body's own collagen production and can be used for volume restoration and skin rejuvenation. When using Sculptra®, the particles are injected into the tissues and recognized by the immune system as foreign bodies. These particles then become walled off and surrounded with collagen, which is responsible for much of the augmentation. It is unique from the other available fillers because it is actually not a dermal filler. It is a generator that produces new collagen.

The injection is in a fanning technique with a 25 or 27 gauge needle. Numbing cream can be placed before injection to make the injections more comfortable.

Scuptra® comes in a powder and reconstituted. The reconstitution is 2–7 days before the anticipated injection treatment with 6 mL bacteriostatic water and allowed to sit. On the day of injection, another 3 mL of lidocaine with epinephrine is added to the vial to make the total diluent volume 9 mL. The liquid in the vial is not what stays as a result. It is use to dissolve the powder and numb the tissue. The liquid is quickly absorbed by the body and the PLLA is what remains under the skin. Depending on the desired level of augmentation, most patients require about three treatments, six weeks apart. Although results can be noticed as early as six weeks after the treatments, the optimal outcome is not noticed until about six months after the procedure.

There is minimal downtime—you may have some bruise marks at the injection site that may last for 7-10 days, but that is it. Other rare complications include the formation of small nodules under the skin, which may have to be treated by a doctor for resolution. Improperly mixed Sculptra® can cause these nodules. If you experience nodules, let your provider know as soon as possible. These are treatable with some minor needle disruption. Patients are encouraged to massage the area throughout the day for the first five days after the procedure. Maximum results may last 18 months to two years after the injections. However, a small degree of patients may see improvements lasting much longer.

The typical cost for a vial of sculpture is about $800. The amount of Sculptra® to get a humble BBL is probably going to cost you at least **$8,000 to $12,000**. To get a large butt the amount of money you would have to spend is not practical for most people. Is is a good alternative for the person who cannot have cannula scars, and is ok getting it done every 2-5 years, plus has a tremendous amount of shmoney to spend. If someone wanted to deny having a BBL and has their own reality show this would be a good treatment for them (just sayin). Most of the world cannot responsibility spent the amount of money required to get and maintain a large BBL with Sculptra®. It can be used effectively to treat a small irregularity in the skin of a butt or a cellulite dimple, but multiple treatments will be needed.

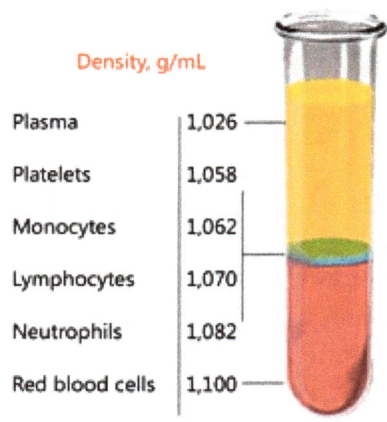

As injecting the amount of filler in the butt is a potentially profitable situation, it is amazing how so many doctors are 'experts' on injecting the butt but probably have done a handful of true BBLs. This product has recently become so popular there is currently a national backorder of it and it isn't available at the time of this chapter being written (we got some, I got the plug).

Truth be told, this is a decent option and the best of the 'off the shelf' fillers for butt augmentation however it can be quite expensive to get yourself a noticeable booty. Vial cost vary per office from $550-$1200. It is a filler that is more expensive compared to the others on the market for the physician to purchase and therefore for the patient to purchase as well.

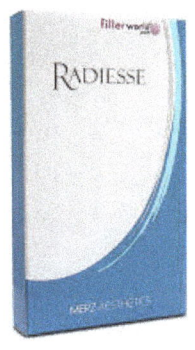

Interestingly, Radiesse®, another filler has now started being used as a body filler. This has been used in the butt as well. It lasts put to 18 months and comes in a larger syringe than most hyaluronic acid fillers. Radiesse® comes in 1.5 cc syringes. Most other fillers come in 1 cc syringes. A cc is the same as a milliliter (ml). A teaspoon can hold 5 cc. When we do BBLs with fat we can inject over 2,000 cc. That would be 2,000 syringes of Juvederm. Most people use 2 syringes in their face! Therefore, a filler that comes from a bottle can never replace a true BBL unless you have unlimited funds like an Armenian family we all know.

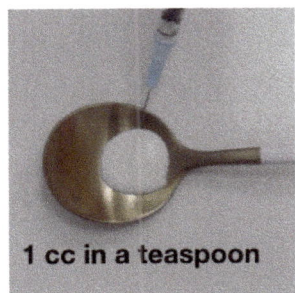

1 cc in a teaspoon

Advantages of fillers vs fat	Disadvantages of fillers
no scars	expensive, not practical for most to achieve a large butt
no lipo needed	can slow to achieve results
little to no downtime	lasts 1-5 years depending on the filler

Advantages of fillers vs fat	Disadvantages of fillers
less risk of severe complications	
no risk of anesthesia	
fast; in and out appointment	

PMMA (polymethyl-methacrylate) is controversial and illegal in countries like Carcas which is punishable by jail time for 2-5 years. It is banned by the FDA in the United States and in Canada. It is still used commonly in Brazil.

These fillers contain about 20 percent of tiny PMMA microspheres (basically acrylic) that are suspended in 80% of purified collagen gel. A few months after it's injected, the collagen gel breaks down and your body produces its own natural collagen to fill out the space under the skin.

These tiny acrylic beads stimulate inner fibrous tissue growth as the human body's natural reaction by our self defense mechanisms to isolate and protect itself against foreign substances. Soft connective tissue strengthening along with PMMA carrier substance can provides instant volume to the buttocks.

The long term risk of PMMA injections may include but are limited to: irregularities of the buttock, lumps at injection sites, disfigurement, and dystrophy of the buttocks. Since it's not FDA approved, it's considered a highly dangerous substance that may result in permanent disfiguration or even DEATH. Patients must know that

PMMA injections for butt augmentation are not only unreliable and costly but also dangerous for your health.

It is not suitable for your butt because it has a very low viscosity. Viscosity is the internal friction of a liquid. Basically if you make a hole in a cup and fill the cut with water it will come out faster than filing the cup up with maple syrup. The unit of measurement used for viscosity is centistokes.
As a reference:

material	viscosity (centipoises)
water	1-5
blood	10
maple syrup	150-200
honey	2,000-3,000
mustard	50,000-70,000
peanut butter	150,000-200,000

Ideally, anything used for butt augmentation must have a viscosity level of more than 3000 centistokes. PMMA injections have a viscosity of 1000 centistokes. This makes it ineffective in buttock enhancement.

There is no doubt that PMMA injections have been found to be effective in treating signs of aging in the face without causing any significant side effects. However, it is not suitable for the butt and can cause many side effects when used for butt enhancement.

I have seen beautiful results with doctors that have used this filler that have lasted more than 10 years and I have seen patients with horrible lumps (granulomas) that required significant surgeries to repair the damage done by this.

In 2018, donated human fat has become available in a syringe. It is sold under the name of Renuva®. There is not actually live fat cells in the filler, instead it is a scaffolding that encourages a patients own fat to replace itself. **Renuva**® provides an off-the-shelf adipose alternative to liposuctioned fat. It is designed to address minor aesthetic defects, such as liposuction irregularities, depressed scars and loss of volume in the hands and cheeks, in a short, in-office procedure. The results from this if it is effective should be very long lasting. According to the website Realself.com a treatment costs $3000. The syringes are sold in 1.5 cc, 3 cc and 5 cc increments. Just as a frame of reference a typical BBL can get again take 2,000 cc of fat injected in it. Therefore, it certainly is not a good alternative for a BBL but instead a small irregularity or depression that you may want repaired.

I don't want to be viewed as a hater that talks smack about something i don't own, but i guess it is going to be inevitable. The idea of Emsculpt® giving a sizable BBL result to me is as crazy as Daddy long neck starting a rap career (athough his one song wasn't as bad as I thought it was going to be).

Emsculpt® has recently hit the market and is being pushed as an alternative to a Brazilian Butt Lift surgery. It is explained that Emsculpt® essentially causes 20,000 muscle contractions in 30 minutes, constricting the muscles beyond any sort of physiological norm, and targeting fat loss to the area of the muscle. Their medical claims include it not only implodes fat cells (for a 19 percent loss after four treatments), but simultaneously builds muscle fibers (by roughly 16 percent) for more defined abs and rounder rear-ends. One company-sponsored study even reported a 10 percent reduction in diastasis recti, the abdominal separation that occurs commonly in pregnancy. This is what they report happens on the stomach.

Magically, (can you sense the sarcasm?) when used on the butt, fat is not destroyed and muscle is stimulated to give you a larger butt. Most of the requests for a butt that I see want more fat on the hips and more projection. There is no muscle on the side of the hips that is capable of being stimulated to grow to fill in the hips. Doing a million squats will certainly build muscle and potentially raise the butt up. It will also burn fat.

Pricing for Emsculpt® varies from practice to practice but we found **$750** to **$1,000** per treatment to be the range. With 4 treatments typically required over 2 weeks, the average total cost for Emsculpt® is **$3,000** to **$4,000**. Emsculpt® is painless and there is no downtime. I personally am not a believer in this, if you can't tell.

There are people out there injecting plasma into the butt to make it grow. Save your money. Plasma is a component of blood and is useless when used to create volume. It will temporarily add volume just as injecting saline under the skin will. Maybe you will get one or two selfies out of it and then it will be absorbed by your body.

PRP is something else. PRP stands for platelet rich plasma. The definition of PRP is autologous plasma that has a platelet concentration well above baseline. While the normal platelet counts in whole blood average 200,000/ml, the platelet counts in PRP should average 1,000,000/ml.

Platelets, also called thrombocytes, develop from the bone marrow. PRP is a concentrated mixture of platelets in plasma, obtained by centrifugation of whole blood. The alpha granules of platelets have growth factors that promote wound healing by promoting angiogenesis and production of extracellular matrix products. These growth factors include platelet-derived growth factor, transforming growth factor-b (TGF-B), vascular endothelial growth factor (VEGF), epithelial growth factor (EGF), insulin-like growth factor, fibroblast growth factor, and platelet-derived angiogenesis factor.

When injected into tissue it does increase the blood supply to the tissue. It has been used for years in the oral and maxillofacial surgery literature and orthopedic literature. Injecting it alone should not increase the amount of fat that will 'grow' in your butt. It is being tested as an additive to the fat that is injected. Like adding some pepper to the soup that is being added.

- In a test tube there has been studies showing it helps and some showing it hurts the growth of fat.
- in animals it has been shown to help fat survival
- in humans it has been shown both to increase fat retention and make no difference

It is still being studied and is inconclusive. I was using this for a while and I am unsure if it really makes a difference in fat retention. I am convinced however, it does help to some degree with post operative pain.

In the face where one injects 50 cc of fat to the cheeks, nasolabial fold, temples or jawline it is an easier argument to inject 5 cc of PRP. But adding 5 cc of PRP to the butt when we are adding 2,500 cc of fat may have the same effect as peeing in a large swimming pool.

Adding PRP alone as a therapy to grow your butt is useless.

SVF stands for stromal vascular fractions. (SVF) is the extracellular matrix products and cells that remain after adipose tissues and fluids are removed from the liposuctioned fat. The SVF is a relatively small proportion of the entire lipoaspirate but is highly enriched in adipose derived stem cells (ASCs) and growth factors.

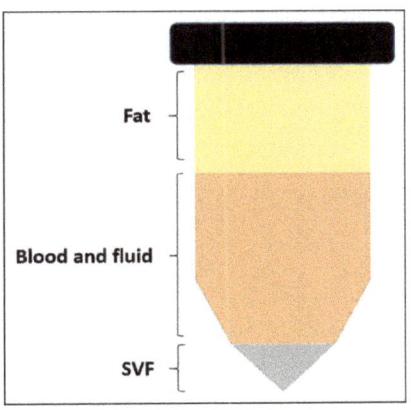

Due to FDA regulations we cannot fully isolate stem cells from fat in this country but even so, reinjecting the very bottom-most portion of liquid of the reinjection slurry could potentially improve fat survival. Injecting SVF alone to gain butt size is not possible in the US or practical in any other country. Stem cells are being isolated for more critical purposes like making vital organs, bring diseases, and repairing tissues. I do not think there will be much resources spent on studying stem cells to make a bigger ass.

I warn patients who are looking for fillers for the cheapest prices, to be careful what you look for because you may find it. There are such low prices some offices are advertising I question the product they are buying. Sites like Groupon and plain old competition are driving prices down so low that there is little to no room for profit by the provider if they are using 'real stuff'. You can get fillers from other countries like Canada or China that are not FDA regulated for mad cheap. I even saw on alibaba.com you can buy fillers! The scary thing is these products can have contaminates that can potentially hurt a patient by disease transmission or complications associated with injections of impure foreign bodies. Fake Botox (Faux tox) is another problem but not the topic for this book. Beware! Real Botox has a hologram on the bottle. Fake Botox does not. Is the price too cheap? Ask to see the bottle! Ask to watch the dilution!

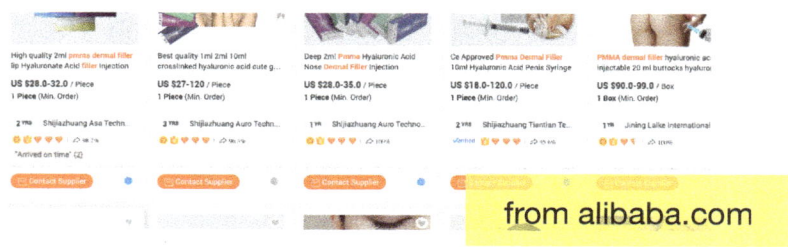

There is a product being tested now called Volup-A that is not yet FDA approved. It is for those who do not have adequate fat to achieve their goals. The filler is essentially microbeads of silicone. This IS NOT a silicone liquid injection. The concept is that these solid silicone beads will encapsulate and prevent migration. It will likely carry the same risks as a fat transfer with regard to fat embolism. Personally, I am going to wait for others to experiment with this before offering it to my patients. A product like this may have long term consequences that we will not learn about until years have passed.

Chapter 13: Silicone butt implants

"Real bitch, only thing fake is the boobs."

Cardi B

This topic can be confusing for patients so let me make myself clear.

I am referring to a silicone implant, not 'shots' of silicone. This is a prefabricated solid piece of silicone that is inserted by an incision.

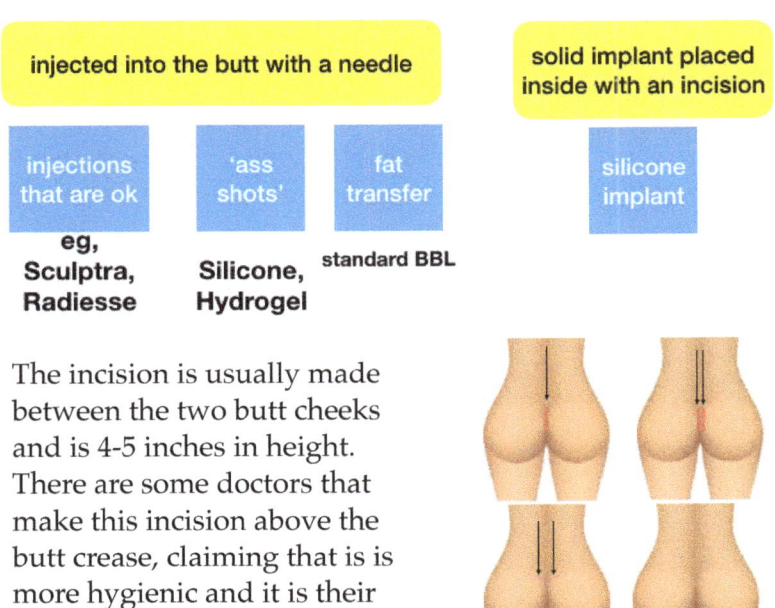

The incision is usually made between the two butt cheeks and is 4-5 inches in height. There are some doctors that make this incision above the butt crease, claiming that is is more hygienic and it is their belief it can cause less chance of infection. The original incision

for this surgery is below the butt fold

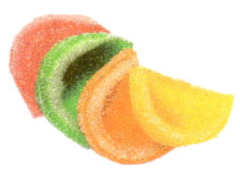

In the United States the only option for materials used are solid silicone elastomer implants. If one were to cut a butt implant in half it would look like the inside of one of those Kosher for passover fruit candies or Jelly rings (left). This is opposed to a breast implant which is a sticky gooey gel (right).

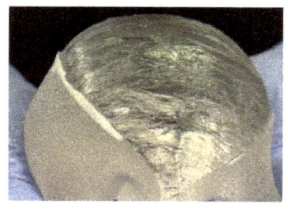

The advantage of these solid implants are that they do not leak, and they maintain their form upon bending unlike the silicone gel implants used in other countries. They are however hard and need to be placed within the muscle to get a nice result. Inside the muscle it has the best protection, least chance of migration, allows the butt to feel softer, less chance of capsular contracture, and less chance of droopy skin.

When choosing the proper implant the variables include:
size
shape (round, anatomical or custom made)
smooth or textured
firmness.

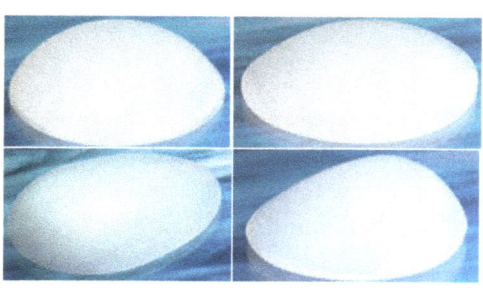

Most people have stayed away from textured implants in the butt because of the scare of textured implants in the breast causing a rare type of cancer. BIA-ALCL is a rare and highly treatable type of lymphoma that can develop around breast implants, most likely from chromic irritation caused by the rough surface of the implant. This is a cancer of the immune system, not a type of breast cancer. The current lifetime risk of BIA-ALCL is estimated to be 1:2,207 - 1:86,029 for women with textured implants based upon current confirmed cases and textured implant sales data past the past two decades. When caught early, BIA-ALCL is usually curable. There have been a report in June 2019 of the same disease process being discovered associated with a textured butt implant in California.

With any butt surgery the most common complaint is, I want it bigger. The nice thing about silicone implants it has the strength to push the skin out in what we call projection. Where sometimes the skin does not expand well enough to fit a soft compressible substance like fat. The beauty of butt implants WHEN DONE CORRECTLY, in comparison to fat transfers are they are they are predictable, permanent, creates good projection, should not cause fat necrosis or fat embolism.

That being said, even an implant has limitations. It is here where patients get into trouble. Pushing a doctor into putting a larger implant that they should. The most important part of this surgery is making sure the entire implant is covered by muscle and closing it up without too much tension. Implants that project 3 cm typically fit within the

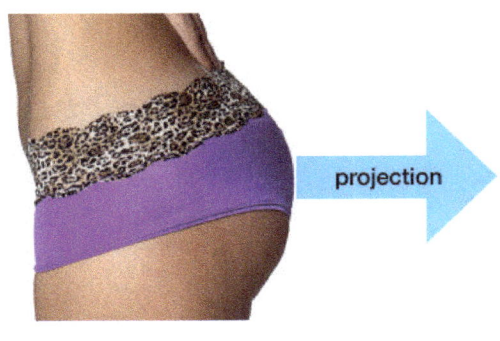

muscle without too much tension. Anything more than that many times you do not know until you are actually doing the procedure. You can place an implant, allow the area to stretch and return for a large implant.

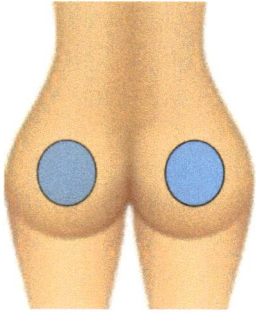

I do not place large implants in the butt on anyone. If I do place an implant it is usually a humble size (less than 300 cc) and comfortably place this in the muscle. Around the area above the muscle I will add fat to further stretch the skin and shape the butt. The implant is really for projection not to fill in the empty spaces on the bottom or sides of the butt. I leave that for fat.

I very rarely place implants in the butt when it is used as a primary source of volume. The complication rate in my opinion is too high for an elective procedure for larger implants. It has been been reported over 30% of these surgeries result in a complication. There is a small group of doctors that are strong advocates of silicone butt implants as a sole source of butt augmentation, some of whom claim a very low complication rate. Based on the mainstream literature, my opinion is not as favorable. If it doesn't sound like a bad idea in theory, let me set it up for you:

1.We have a thin patient who wants a butt with not enough fat for a transfer. Thin out the skin to make room for an implant. Place the implant inside (decreasing the blood supply to the skin). Now spend the majority of your regular day sitting on your ass.
        a)When you apply pressure on your skin, it turns white because the blood supply is diverted away.

So now a compromised site is sitting right on your 'hard' implant further damaging the skin.

    1. Silicone gel implants are not allowed in the US. The rupture rate was reported to be 97%! That shows the amount of pressure is being put on these implants and why breast implants and butt implants are a complete different situation. But from this, we clearly see there is a good amount of weight being placed on the material, stressing its limits.

b. This can affect the scar that was created. Scar tissue made for the incision to get the implant in has a decreased blood supply. Now you are compromising it even more. There is a chance of wound dehiscence (wound break down).

2. Chance of infection. It take 1 million bacteria to contaminate a normal wound to create an infection. It only takes 10,000 bacteria to create an infection on an implant. We are choosing the dirtiest area on the body to place a sterile implant inside. This is not the case for the breast which sterility can be preserved much easier.

3. We are placing a solid implant that is not round like that of breast. If a round breast implant rotates you would have no idea. An anatomical implant for the breast (one made in a teardrop shape) can rotate if the pocket is overly dissected and can require a revision. These are shaped implants in the butt and a shift can be seen through the skin. There is a flatter side to a butt implant and a convex side. If the pocket was made too large during the surgery to fit the implant this cannot be predictably or easily repaired at the time of placement. If the pocket is too large for the implant it can move from its intended position. Or if the implant is in the wrong plane it can shift, flip, or droop. We have all seen the viral video of the girl with the

implant that flips or is hanging off her ass because her skin is too thin to support the implant and it was placed in the wrong plane.

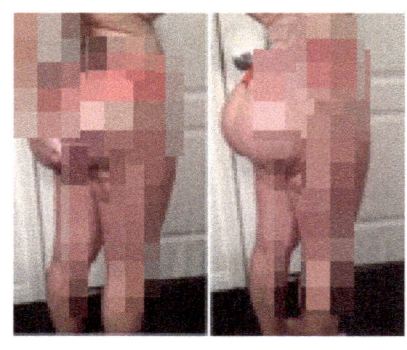

That being said a tasteful small round implant can be placed deep INSIDE the muscle and do quite well. The smaller sized implants are less likely to be felt. They are less likely to put too much tension on the wound and is more likely to close better. They are less likely to see the edges of the implant. A composite butt lift is now becoming more popular where a small implant is placed inside the butt muscle and fat is place over the muscle, around the implant to give the butt a soft feel and nice shape. The beauty of this is in a patient deficient in projection with a tight butt, it will create a nice mound in the muscle to set a frame work to allow the fat to be placed in a nice aesthetic fashion. Some call this a Super Charged BBL.

This hybrid BBL (small implant + fat) gets the projection from the implant, minimizes many of the risks associated with butt implants, and the fat allows one to shape around the implant, hips, and lower butt.

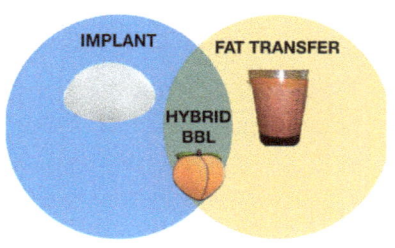

Chapter 14: Butt Shots: Everything you want to know, and everything your NEED to know

Tansar Mir, MD
Board Certified Plastic and Reconstructive Surgeon
www.buttockreconstruction.com

Butt shots or butt injections have had a role in society for over thirty years. They are very common and popular in many cultures and regions, but they are especially popular amongst Blacks and Hispanics. There is an epidemic in this country and throughout South America, in particular Colombia and Venezuela, where currently hundreds of thousands of people, mostly women, but also transgenders and males who attempted to augment their buttocks with injections are suffering complications of these shots and not able to seek appropriate medical or surgical care. These injections are almost always non medical grade silicone and patients also almost never know exactly what was injected into them. Regardless of what is injected, the body reacts to any foreign substance, whether it be silicone, "biopolymers", PMMA, or tire sealant in the same way- and that is to reject it!

In the last 15 years or so, having a bigger booty has been deemed as desirable and this is due to the influences of pop culture. Social media alone and the rise in popularity of Instagram and other photo sharing apps has emphasized beauty and image more so that in the past. People feel a need to compete with others for more followers which in turn can lead to more popularity, endorsements, money, fame and countless opportunities.

Equally important, singers, rappers, actresses, dancers, social media influencers and other "celebrities" have flaunted their asses in art, photo or social media and this alone has made buttock augmentation the fasting growing field in plastic surgery today.

Cardi B, for example has admitted to having these buttock injections. However, MANY other "celebrities" have also had these shots yet they have revealed to the public that they have. Strippers are also a subset of the population that gravitates towards butt shots.

The only safe and approved was to augment your buttocks is fat transfer, aka a Brazilian Butt Lift or buttock implants. There are some legitimate doctors in this country injecting actual Hyaluronic Acid (or a compounded version of it) or Sculptra® for buttock augmentation non-operative PROCEDURES. These are VERY expensive procedures and are also NOT FDA approved and there have been ZERO scientific long term studies proving efficacy or sustained cosmetic results.

What are the common signs and symptoms of complications of butt shots?
1. There are local symptoms such as burning and itching and pain of the buttocks, low back pain, and signs such as skin discoloration/hyperpigmentation, dimpling and soft tissue hardening, lumps and bumps and wounds that breakdown (open wounds) and drain.

2. Systemic symptoms include being tired and fatigued, having shortness of breath, having a stuffy nose, having anxiety, heart palpitations, having pain and numbness of ones hands and legs, having difficulty sitting or walking, having

autoimmune like diseases, being prone to recurrent infections especially of the lungs, buttock and legs (cellulitis), fevers/chills/sweats, having rashes and other skin breakouts or flare ups.

This begs the question- Whose fault is it when patients get complications from these butt shots???

One can blame the injectors, who in America are NEVER real doctors. It's usually an esthetician or a "Doctor" from another country or some random person and the procedure usually takes place in the black market. Black market means in an underground marketplace, often hotel rooms, spas, someone's house or pop-up clinics. The injector usually travels from city to city and often times becomes unreachable if a complication arises. Injecting more than the tiniest syringe of MEDICAL GRADE SILICONE for eye surgery is NOT FDA approved or regulated. Doctors and plastic surgeons are not the ones doing these injections and moreover, they have ZERO training on these shots and the consequences of them. These fake practitioners who perform these butt shots also have no malpractice insurance and rarely can be held financially liable to lawsuits especially because its a cash transaction and the money usually gets hidden or spent. Some injectors have been prosecuted by law when patients have died but that's of no use to the victim.

You can also make the argument that there are a lot of doctors, especially plastic surgeons in this country who refuse to treat patients who got butt shots and rather choose to chastise them and say these patients are getting what they deserve. While I TOTALLY DISAGREE with this statement, there is some validity to it. I mean, if someone told you to meet them at a hotel on a certain day, instructed you not to tell anyone, ask you to bring cash to meet someone coming in from another city, then promise you no complications and then put a NEEDLE in your ass with some unknown product that you can't verify while NOT having you sign a consent form and NOT showing you and professional medical degrees or certificates, and you go back multiple times for additional sessions- wouldn't this sound alarms in your head that something shady is happening???

Here's some secret inside information. The reason that a majority of plastic surgeons refuse to treat butt shot patients who develop complications is because **THEY DO NOT KNOW HOW TO**. There is ZERO education on this topic in medical school, minimal literature in the journals, and most have NEVER done this operation or seen it done or have any experience with it. Also, once a doctor operates on someone, they assume liability for the patient from that day on, which kind of absolves the injector and any previous people who treated or touched the patient and that is NOT something any well trained plastic surgeon wants to take on.

Why do people get butt shots?

Ok, let's talk about the appeal of butt shots, as told to me by hundreds of patients (disclaimer: I am **NOT** endorsing butt shots; rather, I am CONDEMING them):

1. They are relative cheap (approximately $1000-1500 a session) as opposed to a BBL which is at least $10,000.
2. There is no no need for anesthesia as opposed to BBL or buttock implants which usually require general or spinal anesthesia.
3. They provide instantaneous "results" or inflation of the buttocks and hips.

4. There is zero recovery or time off work. BBLs require you not to lay or sit for approximately 3-4 weeks.
5. The ability to do more sessions relatively easily to get you exactly the size you want and "fill"any dents or concavities you don't like.
6. Most people who have had the shots done know someone else who had it done and are told "they are doing fine" and without any problems so everyone thinks that they too will be fine. People also have a sense of invincibility and never think that anything bad will happen to them.
7. To do a BLL , you MUST have some fat to transfer. So if you're skinny and have no excess fat, what the heck can you transfer to your buttocks that will make any substantial cosmetic difference? Nothing, so some skinnier patients use this excuse to justify their butt shots.

Why shouldn't you get butt shots?
Now let's talk about the negatives of butt shots, and unfortunately this is what matters the most!

1. The human body is very smart. It knows what belongs in the body and what doesn't. When some large amount of silicone (or any foreign material) is injected into your body, it will mess up your immune system. Your body will start attacking itself and it WILL lead to numerous signs and symptoms. ASIA syndrome, or any other type of autoimmune disease is very highly correlated with butt shots.

2. Most people who have had butt shots will likely have symptoms or signs at some point, but they may not recognize why. Lots of people who had the shots themselves don't correlate the shots with their sickness and many times are not honest or forthcoming to their doctors about their history of receiving illegal buttock injections. Moreover, most doctors themselves won't be able to infer that your illness stems from these shots so lots of times people end up getting excessive and expensive workups and medical testing without any definitive diagnosis or proper treatment. Many butt shot patients get started on antibiotics and steroids, both of which can have harmful side effects on their bodies.

3. Getting these shots is like a ticking time bomb! Although someone you know had the shots previously and are doing "fine", it does NOT mean they are free and clear. I have seen patients develop complications as early as a few days after the shots to 30 years later. I don't think anyone would want to live with this knowledge in the back of their head.

4. It is IMPOSSIBLE to remove ALL of the silicone or whatever was injected into your buttocks or hips or breasts or face or legs. We have invented a staged protocol where we have successfully removed a very large percentage of the foreign material (and the associated dead tissue it caused) in patients who were very sick or showed signs of soft tissue and/ or skin necrosis.

5. We do NOT remove the silicone in patients who do NOT have symptoms or whose bodies don't show

signs of rejection or necrosis so it's not as easy as returning a dress to the store if you don't like it. You are stuck with it and your body will likely get ruined in time and will cost you way more in health problems and finances and regret and time off work that you could ever imagine. So my point is, if you are contemplating getting these shots, DON'T. Instead RUN far away from them. Furthermore, if you want to be a good samaritan, then you should report the injector to the local authorities so you can save other people's lives!

6. You CAN die from these shots. Death usually occurs really early or really late. If some of the injected material gets in a vein at the time of your injections and goes to your heart and lungs, you can die. This is what happens when you read stories in the newspaper about people who died within days of their injections. You can also die much later than the time of injections if your tissues get infected, necrotic, the wounds open up and you get sepsis. This requires emergent surgery attempting to save lives and often times leads to limb loss and inevitable death!

Is it possible to remove the silicone and what surgery does that?

The ONLY effective way to "remove" a lot of the silicone is through open surgery from a surgeon who is extremely familiar with the disease and has extensive experience in this operation and one that is aware of complications that can arise and takes steps to minimize any potential complications. Again, it is IMPOSSIBLE to remove all of the silicone but an experienced surgeon can remove enough of it to restore your health.

Accurate, real, unfiltered before and after photos of patients with similar body habitus/stage of necrosis are critical to see so a patient can have a realistic expectation of what their cosmetic outcome may look like. If anyone shows you only amazing photos, that should raise a red flag.

I have yet to perfect this surgery in terms of producing the best cosmetic outcome while restoring health and minimizing complications, but I probably have the most experience in terms of doing this surgery, knowledge of common and rare complications, performing these in hospital settings only with constant supervision, taking on the most difficult cases that were referred by doctors from all of over the country (and internationally), and successfully restoring the health of approximately 98% of patients!

These surgeries often cause significant blood loss during the operations and many patients end up getting blood transfusions. This surgery should NEVER be performed in any setting where there is not adequate staff and physicians to monitor and to provide backup support GOD forbid a rare complication occurs. Remember, the goal of the removal surgery is to RESTORE HEALTH and get you to heal.

Acceptable cosmetic outcome is also important but this surgery is so complex and requires such large amounts of debridement or removal that often time patients are left with long and uneven scars and a flatter appearing buttock.

Can I get liposuction to remove the silicone?

For those of you who had the butt shots and thinking about liposuction to "remove" the silicone or a BBL to add healthy tissue to the area, DO NOT do it. People who get the shots are obviously very focused on appearance and some cultures value beauty at all costs and people don't want big scars or the potential cosmetic disfigurement that open surgery techniques may lead to. Thus, some people end up getting liposuction or "laser lipo" to TRY to remove it which DOES NOT WORK. Liposuction techniques involve cannulas and these create tunnels and pathways for the silicone to migrate to other parts of your body, especially your legs/knees/ankles as well as to your groin and private area and up your back. Liposuction not only will cost you money and comes with inherent risks itself (from anesthesia, or fat emboli), it will NOT alleviate any of your symptoms and will cause further, progressive, IRREVERSIBLE side effects over the course of the rest of your life.

What if I get a BBL to add healthy tissue to my butt instead of having open surgery to remove it?

BBLs to add healthy tissue are another faulty idea propagated by some cosmetic surgeons and something that butt shot patients who are not ready for a flatter buttock seek. We STRONGLY recommend against this. It does ZERO in terms of removal of the silicone and furthermore, it actually feeds the autoimmune process in a negative way. What happens inside your body after the shots, is that the fat and muscle and skin eventually necrose, or die. So doing a BBL just adds more fuel to the fire. You're adding more fat that the silicone will contaminate and eventually die.

What are my options for reconstruction after silicone removal?

So you have the removal surgery and now you want a big butt again. What are your options for buttock reconstruction? We recommend that you wait at least 6 months for any minor surgical revisions such as dog ear removal, and wait at least 9 months from the removal for a BBL if you qualify for one. By qualify I mean, you healed without any complications such as a large seroma or got an infection, you waited enough time for the tissues to soften, and you have enough donor fat in our body to transfer to your buttocks. We also perform a "buttock lift" at the time of your removal surgery and sometimes perform an advanced lift where you use some of your excess skin and dunk it in or "fold it" to autoaugment your buttocks- this is done 1 year after the removal surgery if your tissues softened.

What if I had butt shots and am not ready or not a candidate for removal. Any tips, Doc?

Some people think vigorous exercise will help them but this is contrary to what we have found. We recommend that you cease any and all high impact exercise since this causes the material to migrate to you back, groins, private area, and legs. We only recommend yoga and pilates as low-impact sources of exercise.

The people who have gotten the butt shots also inherently want to flaunt their asses so they spend a lot of time on beaches and tanning. We have found that the sun, hot tubs, saunas, tanning salons and other hot activities actually speeds up the discoloration of your skin, which is usually irreversible. So we thus strongly recommend any tanning or exposure to the sun or hot environments.

CONCLUSION

By now, you should realize that butt shots are illegal and only performed in the black market for a reason- and that is because they are unsafe and DEADLY. If you are thinking about increasing the size of your butt, you should consult with a cosmetic or plastic surgeon and explore if you are a candidate for a BBL or buttock implants. You should RESIST the temptation to fall into the trap of thinking you are invincible or convince yourself that since someone you know had the illegal shots and appear to be doing fine with an amazing result that those results are reproducible or final. They are NOT.

Those people likely will have complications at some point in their lives, end up needing many surgeries over many years, will spend tons of money, miss many weeks of school or work and have extended time away from their families or loved ones, and may end up with a deformed buttock to top it off.

I wish that I could say that I will never perform another silicone removal surgery (because the epidemic went away), but that will not be the case. There are hundreds of thousands of people in this country and abroad who have been VICTIMS of illegal buttock injections and will need our services to RESTORE THEIR HEALTH. While the removal and reconstructive surgeries are extremely complex, work intensive and require very close monitoring post-operatively, we find these surgeries to be incredibly rewarding with an extremely high personal satisfaction in being able to restore patients' health and allow them to live normal lives and return to being mothers or fathers and being able to meaningfully contribute to society.

If I can help, do not hesitate to contact me @ tmirmd.com
(212) 606 8150

Chapter 15: The FDA and their 'approval'

"I bet you I can make that ass hot. C'mon bae, drop it like an ass shot"

Childish Gambino

If a treatment is FDA approved, does it work better?

What is the FDA?
This is off the FDA website,
" The Food and Drug Administration is responsible for protecting the public health by ensuring the safety, efficacy, and security of human and veterinary drugs, biological products, and medical devices; and by ensuring the safety of our nation's food supply, cosmetics, and products that emit radiation."

Long story short, it is a government agency that makes sure the potential benefit of a medical device/drug outweighs the risk of it. It does not mean that it has been tested by the FDA themself to prove that it is effective as a treatment. It only means enough data has been presented to them that the harm is relatively less than the potential benefit.

So if someone says, "this item is FDA approved for cellulite". This does not necessary mean it has achieved the holy grail of results. Instead, it means if done properly to treat cellulite, the harm from this therapy is minimal.

ELIGIBLE	NOT ELIGIBLE
drugs, vaccines, cellular therapies, and blood and blood products.	compounded drugs (made in a pharmacy)
medical devices	perfumes, makeup, moisturizers, shampoos, hair dyes, face and body cleansers, and shaving preparations
	dietary supplements

Items in the cosmetic surgery world will fall into one of 4 categories with regard to the FDA:
A. Approved for a specific use [i.e., labeled and approved by the U.S. Food and Drug Administration (FDA) for marketing
B. Approved and permitted for off-label use (i.e., legal use of an FDA-approved product
outside of the clinical indications of the product labeling)
C. Non-approved (i.e., not approved by the FDA for any purpose, and thus ineligible for
off-label use
D. not eligible for FDA approval

Just because something is being used 'off label' does not mean its use is forbidden. You as a patient should be told by your doctor or provider that the product is off label but there are many products that you probably were not aware of are being used 'off label'. Examples are:
    a. Botox was only FDA approved for severe frown lines in 2002, Since then it has been approved to make moderate to severe frown lines, crow's feet and forehead

lines better. It still is used off label in the lips, neck, masseter (jaw muscles), and depressor angular oris (frowning muscles)

    b. in the world of breast surgery many times implants are associated with 'off label use' including:
        1. including closed capsulotomy
        2. iodophor pocket irrigation
        3. implant overfill and underfill,
        4. endoscopically assisted augmentation
        5. Silicone implants being used on patients under the age of 22
        6. Using Singulair to treat capsular contracture

The FDA classifies medical devices as either Class I, II or III devices. Each class has different regulations and are monitored differently.

I	Class I devices are subject to the least regulatory control	gloves, toothbrush, bandages	Class I devices are generally exempt from the regulatory process and can be marketed without receiving clearance from the FDA. The only requirement is that manufacturers of Class I devices register their establishment and list their generic products with the FDA

II	medical devices are more complicated than Class I devices and present a higher category of risk because they are more likely to come into sustained contact with a patient.	blood pressure vuff, syringes, contact lenses, gloves	Technically, Class II devices are less risky and can be reviewed under 510(k). However, some risky devices are determined to be Class II because their manufacturers can demonstrate that they are "substantially equivalent" to another device that is already on the market.
III	"usually sustain or support life, are implanted or present a potential unreasonable risk of illness or injury."	pacemakers, breast implants, defibrillaotrs, replacement hart saves	Most Class III devices must undergo a stringent PMA process, which requires clinical and laboratory studies, and extensive data, including information on manufacturing processes.

To make you an FDA genius I just want to clarify one last important distinction.

The two main ways to get the FDA to allow medical devices to be marketed in the US are either

1. Premarket approval which requires clinical and laboratory studies to determine safety and efficacy (5% of devices use this route)

2. 510 K which requires no clinical trials and little oversight (90% of the devices use this route)

There are various subtypes under these two categories

Other routes to FDA approval include

3. de novo - used when a device is low risk and there is nothing similar to it done before (like you invented the first toothbrush)

4. humanitarian device exemption - it used to help encourage companies to invent devices that help conditions affecting fewer than 4,000 people in the US per year.

5. product development protocol - This method is generally used if the device has already undergone clinical testing and has been approved in a country with established medical device regulations.

6. custom device exemption - used for prescription glasses, customized dental devices

7. expanded access option - this allows a investigational device to be used on a seriously ill person with few or any other options

The most popular route for FDA approval and the largest amount of recalls happen in the category of 501k approval.

If a company can prove its device is "substantially equivalent" to another already on the market, it can skip clinical trials and testing. This saves a company millions of dollar and much time. Unlike the more rigorous PMA standard, which is to reasonably ensure safety and effectiveness, the 510(k) standard is to determine whether a device is substantially equivalent to a legally marketed device.

In summary, when the FDA clears a device through 510(k), it is not examining if the product is safe or effective for use in patients. It is agreeing with the maker's claim that the device is similar to another device already on the market

In federal law it states that 510(k) clearance "does not in any way denote official approval of the device." Any representation that creates the impression that the FDA has officially approved a product with 510(k) clearance is considered misleading and is illegal.

How does this relate to the butt?
Solid gluteal implants, along with calf implants and pectoral implants, were marketed as "solid silicone carving blocks," like the facial silicone implants that have been used for many years. They were classified as Class II devices with a 510(k) Premarket Notification authorizing their use in the United States.

Just recently, some companies have begun to market these devices specifically as gluteal implants, and implants specific for certain body parts.

FYI, silicone gel implants (like for the breast), however, are not covered by this notification and remain classified as Class III devices that can be used only in conformity with the FDA's strict requirements for this class of products.

Chapter 16: Getting ready for surgery, and the perfect candidate

"Curvy little body, love your surface."
A Boogie wit da Hoodie

The perfect patient for a BBL is someone who is healthy, has a nice amount of fat but not obese, skin on the butt that is loose, an exaggerated lower back curve, someone who is mentally strong, has a good support system at home, has time to recover, and is realistic and patient with their expectations. If you possess all of the above, PLEASE call ME!

This is a difficult surgery to recover from. The injection into the butt is not painful but to get extreme results in the waistline you have to be aggressive with liposuction. You can see advertisements on 'lunchtime lipo' all this other nonsense, most of which is just marketing and disingenuous in what to expect. To get gorgeous results one must go HAM[2] with lipo. This results in pain, a drop in hemoglobin, a drop in blood pressure, dizziness, headaches.

It is often taxing to sleep, and difficult to go to the bathroom. You cannot sit for an extended amount of time. All of these challenges are addressed in other chapters in depth. In summary, you should be healthy enough to handle this challenge to your body.

Looking back at the results of my patients, the most commonly requested description in size is

---

[2] HAM= hard as a mofo

- i want to look natural
- match with my legs
- not Black Chyna big (sorry Black Chyna, *who refused to write my intro btw*)

To accomplish this for most people the BMI should be 25-28. Too little may limit the size of the butt, too high a BMI may result in a large amount of redundant loose skin. If the skin is overstretched from being overweight, the loose skin occurs like taking the air out of a balloon. The fat normally supported the skin, but now the empty sack remains. This is a broad generalization, and the individual plan for you should be discussed with your doctor. Ask your doctor, what should my weight be before surgery to give me the best result? It may be something that he or she has not even thought about.

People that were heavier in their life often have looser skin in their butt. However this not always the case. If you have tight skin back there, there is not much you can do to stretch it out. Many spas have suction cup devices that claim to stretch the skin out. I do believe suction to the skin will stretch the skin, but the suction would have to be in place 24/7 for a few weeks. Something not very realistic. This has been studied in the orthopedic literature as the functional matrix theory. Form follows function. Meaning, applying the pulling (or sucking pressure) on the skin will cause the skin to grow. An hour treatment in the spa will not likely make a difference in my opinion aside from some temporary swelling.

This surgery is not easy to recover from. This surgery is not cheap. This surgery is best when it's done once, done right, and finished. Do you part. Come at the recommended weight. It may be adding a few pounds and it may be losing a few. I can't tell you how many times I have this conversation with patients. I tell them to loose 20 pounds, and they gain 10. Many people think since they are having surgery, the doctor can just suck it out. It doesn't always work like this. It can also compromise how your skin behaves after its support has been removed.

Chapter 17: Anesthesia options

"I be getting high just to balance out the lows."
                                                    Drake

The fat injections into the butt are not very uncomfortable however the liposuction part can be. Here are all the anesthesia options:

1. Local anesthesia (tumescent anesthesia)
2. Oral sedation (PO sedation)
3. iv sedation
4. general anesthesia
5. spinal anesthesia

It is pretty much universally agreed upon that the anesthesia involved will include at least some form of tumescent anesthesia. So some doctors go with tumescent alone, while others go with tumescent and options 2, 3, 4 or 5.

More of an explanation about tumescent anesthesia can be found in the next chapter. It is essentially a combination of different drugs (numbing medications included) mixed in a fluid and then injected into the fat. A small incision is made and a blunt tip cannula (metal tube with multiple holes) and the fluid is injected into the tissue.

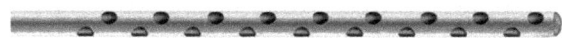

The fluid should be warmed.

1. This is because it helps maintain body temperature of the patient. During surgery a patients ability to regulate their own temperature becomes affected and they have a hard time staying warm. It is almost like the patient becomes cold blooded (much like a reptile) during surgery. The temperature of the patient needs to be kept warm by warm tumescent fluid, warm iv fluid, warming blankets, a warm room and they even have warming mattress that go under the patient on the table.
2. The other reason is it helps minimize blood loss. The body stops bleeding by activating what is called the coagulation cascade. There are heat sensitive proteins in the cascade that work best when the body is warm.

IV sedation:
With iv sedation, the patient is on the monitor with an anesthesia provider watching the vitals signs of the patient. 3 stickers are on your chest monitoring the heart. A sticker or a clip on your finger monitors how much oxygen is in the blood. A blood pressure cuff is on the arm. A small tube is placed near the mouth or nose to measure the amount of carbon dioxide the patient is breathing out. A temperature probe is often placed on the patient's forehead to monitor their temperature. Sometimes a BIS monitor is placed on the patient's forehead. This is an EEG, which measures brainwaves and tells the provider deep the patient is during sedation. This is not a requirement but is an extra tool that is useful to monitor 'how deep of a sleep' the person is having. For the patients who are scared of "waking up" during

surgery, this is some extra reassurance to make sure there is no memory of the surgery.

The patient during iv sedation is breathing on their own. There are 3 different depths of iv sedation:

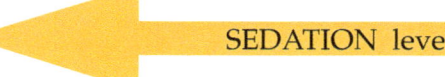
SEDATION level

This is described in the chart shown below:

	min sedation	moderate/ conscious sedation	deep sedation	General anesthesia
responsiveness	nml	verbal or tactile stimulation	to repeated painful stimuli	unresponsive to painful stimuli
airway	nml	no intervention needed	intervention may be required	intervention usually required
breathing spontaneously	nml	adequate	may be inadequate	usually inadequate
cardiovascular function	nml	normal	usually maintained	may be impaired

Levels of sedation can also be accomplished by giving oral medication. This can be quite dangerous as well. Many doctors may underestimate the intensity of the drug, and in the outcome, can give too much. The effect is not seen right away and takes time to 'kick in'. You do not want to give too much. Also, because there is no iv hooked up one may ignore the need for monitors and the patient can be deeper than expected. Because there is no iv access if some intervention needs to take place, such as a reversal medication, it is not readily available.

When the depth of sedation goes deep and the patient no longer responds to painful stimuli and breathing likely requires assistance, a level of general anesthesia has now been achieved.

General anesthesia has the same monitors described above with some other non invasive monitors. A breathing tube is generally placed to support the airway and a ventilator is used to maintain breathing during the surgery while under general anesthesia.

Spinal anesthesia is used rarely but can be used to anesthetize the areas planned for liposuction. A local anesthesia is injected first between the vertebrae allowing for the needle to enter the space for injection. When done correctly the patient should be completely numb in the areas being treated. Sounds great. So why isn't this done more regularly. This procedure is not without risks to the spinal cord.

Additionally, the provider can:
1. miss the block completely - and it does not work, so now what? You need a back up plan.
2. The block can be incomplete - only a portion of the area is anesthetized
3. The block can wear off mid procedure

4. The block can migrate up, can potentially affect the patient's ability to breathe on their own and breathing may need to be assisted.

If it is effective the offset of numbness can be quite long and the patient would likely have to sit in recovery long after what is a routine recovery time.

What is my philosophy with anesthesia for liposuction and why?

I perform tumescent anesthesia with general anesthesia almost exclusively for my liposuction cases. This is why:

1. Results

Even though I do use tumescent (numbing fluid) into the area before doing liposuction, to get impressive results I need to be aggressive with liposuction. That is the only way to really created a snatched waist. At some point the liposuction fluid will be sucked out and fat may still remain. When a patient is squirming around on the operating table in discomfort, it is very hard to operate. Mentally, for me, I cannot continue to work on someone if I know I am hurting them. Additionally, the patient may jump around if they are uncomfortable, and can be injured with the liposuction cannula by an inadvertent movement resulting in an injury to a critical organ, deep to the correct liposuction plane.

2. Safety

As mentioned above, in order to get beautiful results one needs to be aggressive with liposuction. It is in my opinion to be able to keep someone comfortable with local anesthesia alone and still do a good job. One of the most common causes of death during liposuction is from a lidocaine overdose. Although using lidocaine with tumescent has a wide margin of safety, when a patient is uncomfortable it is my belief some of these overdoses were not from miscalculations or lack of information, but from an effort of trying to make the patient comfortable when the maximum amount of lidocaine has already been achieved. This can cause nerve, brain, and heart toxicity and can have very significant repercussions if not recognized and treated quickly. Liposuction was banned in Florida because of an increasing number of deaths years ago, the cause of deaths were mostly lidocaine overdoses (too much numbing medications).

Another concern that sounds counterintuitive, is the safety of being awake, not only reacting by physically moving during the surgery but the vital signs of a person. When someone is in pain, their heart rate and blood pressure can become elevated. Such a period of elevated vital signs depending on the severity can lead to heart arrhythmias and even something as severe as a stroke. Having someone asleep with intravenous access and monitoring their vital signs medications can be administered to modify these parameters and ensure a patients safety.

Can liposuction be performed awake? Yes. In my hands I do not feel comfortable with a large liposuction case doing this awake. A small amount with ample numbing fluid can be done but these cases are rare in my office.

Please do not believe any 'hype' about lunchtime lipo or these other silly marketing ploys that are disingenuous. Liposuction is a surgery. Even though there are not huge scars across your body, under the skin surface a very significant surgery took place. These can result in low blood pressure after surgery, bleeding, and bruising.

"You don't know what you don't know" unknown

While I hope most doctors have good intentions, I am aware that there are some who may not. Be cautious being pushed into an option you may not be comfortable with.

For example,
In NY State, if you want to do liposuction and intend on having liposuction in someone's office;
the surgeon can only:
- remove 500 cc (ml) of fat
- cannot use sedation more than minimal sedation (so essentially awake)

UNLESS....
the office is accredited by one of three agencies.

Therefore, you may be misled down a path of local anesthesia because the office where the surgery was to take place may not be accredited. To achieve and maintain accreditation is very labor intensive and expensive. Many offices do not want to be bothered. Additionally, by doing it awaken less staff is needed (no nurse, no anesthesiologist, etc) the doctor saves money by not having to pay this staff. I would like to think most doctors have the patients best interests guiding them but there are some who probably do not. Please keep this in mind when 'price shopping'. When a price is too low, something in your care is being 'cut'.

Chapter 18: Liposuction techniques

"She was supposed to buy your shorty Tyco with your money, she went to the doctor, got lipo with your money."
Kanye West

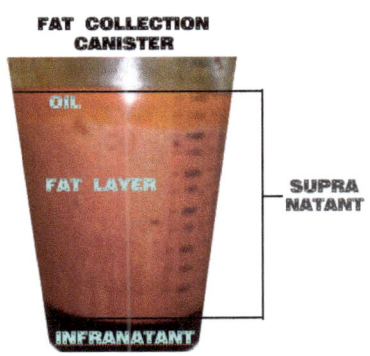

The maximum amount of fat that can be removed in 1 sitting of liposuction is 5 liters (5000 ml or 5000 cc). This is a law in the state of New York (and some others)and is an excellent guideline for the upper limits of safety. 5 liters is a lot of fat. When you look at a canister of liposuction aspirate the fat floats to the the top of the container. The fat is called the supernatant. That is what makes up the 5 liter number. It is not the total amount in the container it is the top portion which is made up of fat and above that you can often see another thin layer of oil from fat cells that were damaged during aspiration.

Doing liposuction beyond 5 liters is called megaliposuction and is very dangerous.

Most patients do not have 5 liters of fat to remove during lipo 360. It's kinda f'd up when doctors write on an IG post 5 liters of fat removed and show someone who is medium sized. I would like to give them the benefit of the doubt but I REALLY doubt 5 liters were removed. Why say 5 liters was removed when it wasn't? Because if the patient complains that more fat was left, the doctor can say, "I took out all I could".

Why is this bad? Well for one, lying to a patient is always bad. But patients who are relatively skinny who don't have 5 L of fat may want to leave the country for surgery, thinking they will get a better result elsewhere. 5 Liters is a lot of fat. If you have more fat than this, it should be done in 2 visits or even better, lose more weight before surgery.

It is generally agreed upon that tumescent anesthesia is the standard of care in liposuction surgery. That is when the numbing solution is injected in the tissue under the skin to allow for safe removal of the fat by liposuction.
The most important aspect of tumescent liposuction is that a local anesthetic is used over a wide area to provide numbing and pain control, using a sufficient quantity of lidocaine far in excess of the conventional dosage. Conventional teaching has widely regarded, that the safe upper limit for lidocaine administration is 7 mg/kg body weight.

Jeffery Klein, a dermatologist from Seattle, showed that in tumescent anesthesia, much higher doses, even up to 45–55 mg/kg weight can safely be administered. This is because in tumescent anesthesia, the rate of absorption of lidocaine is slow, leading to smaller peak values and hence, lesser toxicity. For those who have a scientific interest, the reasons for the slow absorption of lignocaine are:

i. Subcutaneous fat has a low volume of blood flow.
ii. lidocaine is lipophilic, meaning it is easily absorbed by fat.
iii. Diluted epinephrine in saline solution ensures vasoconstriction, thus, minimizing systemic absorption of the lidocaine and decreases bleeding.
iv. The large volume of tumescent solution itself compresses blood vessels by hydrostatic pressure.
v. The very low dilution of lidocaine in Klein's solution does not achieve the gradient required for systemic absorption.
vi. Most of the solution is removed during aspiration, minimizing the duration for absorption.

This slow absorption from subcutaneous fat is like a slow release capsule, with the fat itself acting as the capsule.

What are the different types of liposuction used?

This is coming from a doctor that at one point for a short time used laser liposuction, tried Vaser liposuction, did manual liposuction and now exclusively uses PAL. There are very dishonest and misleading things that I have read on a simple google search comparing smart lipo to regular lipo, and the author coincidentally always paints a picture of the best results for the device they own. I literally saw an advertisement that Smart lipo made small holes and had 3 days downtime, while traditional lipo had 2 weeks of recovery with large scarred holes. This is inaccurate and self serving. What I write below is a neutral assessment based on fact. If it is my opinion from experience I want to share, I will identify it as such.

All liposuction shares some common features. Small holes are made in the skin to allow for the introduction of long metal cannulas into these holes to suck fat out. The recovery is about a week to go make to your routine. Working out should not be done for 6 weeks. This is true for all the different types of liposuction listed below. If you are getting your but done with the liposuction you should give yourself at least 2 weeks to recover.

SAL (suction assisted liposuction) remains the most common modality for liposuction. As stated above, it is considered "traditional liposuction," in which variable-size cannulas are employed, with an external source of suction for removal of fat.

PAL (power assisted liposuction) involves an external power source driving the cannula, which are variable in size and flexible, in a 2-mm reciprocating motion at rates of 4000 cycles per minute. Advocates of PAL contend that it is best used for large volumes, fibrous areas, and revision liposuction. Most people use the Microaire machine and they have a patent on the back and forth vibrating motion of the cannula. Other machines have variations such as a side to side motion to get around the patent. Microaire seems to however have the market on PAL. PAL is definitely ideal to prevent surgeon fatigue and has been shown in the medical literature to have slightly less pain than other modalities (not grossly significant).

UAL (ultrasound assisted liposuction) utilizes ultrasound energy to break down fat and allow removal. Its mechanism of action is primarily mechanical in nature, but cavitation and even thermal effects may occur. With this technique, fat is emulsified, which allows removal through traditional liposuction cannulas. Advantages include less surgeon fatigue, as well as improved results in fibrous areas and in secondary procedures. Disadvantages have been reported to include larger incisions, longer operative times, and the possibility of thermal injury. Management of the UAL probe is essential to preventing thermal injury to the superficial dermis; hence, skin protectors are often employed. This is Vaser liposuction. These devices have a higher incidence of seromas after surgery (what's a seroma? Read Chapter 24)

LAL (laser assisted liposuction) like Smart Lipo has been at the forefront of marketing hype for the past several years. The treatment involves insertion of a laser fiber via a small skin incision. Depending on the manufacturer, the fiber may either be housed within a cannula or stand alone. The most popular player is certainly SMART lipo. The reason this is a household name is they were first to market, just like a photocopy is called a xerox, a photo was called a Polaroid, Acetaminophen is referred to as Tylenol, and a tissue is called Kleenex. They were smart in their marketing, marketing directly to the consumer creating a desire by doctors who were looking to satisfy what they perceived to be a growing need. There are several commercially available lasers on the market under different trade names. The most common available wavelengths in the United States are 924/975 nm, 1064 nm, and 1319/1320 nm. These are some other laser lipo machines that are similar separated by the wavelength of laser and the waveform:

pulsed	1064 nm Nd:YAG	Lipolite- Syneron
continuous	980 nm Diode	Lipotherme – MedSurge Advances Smoothlipo – Eleme
pulsed	1320 nm ND:YAG	CoolTouch –CoolLipo
pulsed	1064/1319 nm ND:YAG	Prolipo- Scition
pulsed	1064 nm/1320 nm Nd:YAG	SMART Lipo – Cynosure
continuous	924/975 nm Diode	SLIM Lipo: Palomar

The laser fiber acts to disrupt fat cell membranes and emulsify fat. Evacuation then commences via traditional liposuction cannulas. If a BBL or other fat transfer was planned the laser would not be used before fat removal because it will damage the fat.

Currently, these devices are being heavily marketed for purported skin-tightening effects. The belief is that the heating of the subdermal tissue may in fact be the contributing factor for LAL's possible skin tightening effect. No large, prospective trials have been undertaken to examine the benefits of LAL over existing technologies, so unfortunately, most of the reports remain anecdotal. A previously published randomized, double-blinded, controlled study by Prado et al showed no difference in the outcomes of LAL versus traditional SAL. In that study, each patient served as his or her own control. Factors evaluated included cosmetic result, postoperative pain, length of operation, and free fatty acids. Besides the lack of difference in the cosmetic outcome of LAL versus SAL, the authors also reported a longer operative time with LAL, less early postoperative pain with LAL, and elevated free fatty acids/triglycerides in the laser-treated lipoaspirate.

A shift in thinking is now happening towards leaving the fat removal to liposuction and the skin tightening to another device. These procedures are done at the same lipo as the liposuction and the device inserted through the liposuction holes.

J-Plasma® (Renuvion®) by Bovie uses cold helium gas combined with low RF energy to create plasma energy that immediately tightens the fibrous support tissue beneath the skin and promotes new collagen formation over time.

BodyTite® by InMode utilizes bi-polar RF energy that can both destroy fat cells and tighten the skin as well as the fibrous network beneath the skin. The skin actually passes like the meat of a sandwich with the device being the bread. A probe is outside the skin and the energy is directed from under the skin to the outside.

Both devices have a similar outcome. They help the skin stick to the deeper layers of tissue, giving the appearance of tighter skin. I do believe J plasma is better (disclaimer: and that is why I own it).

Chapter 19: Hemoglobin and anemia - who cares?

"Hollywood's bleeding, vampires feedin', darkness turns to dust. Everyone;'s gone but no one's leavin."
Post Malone

This chapter is more for the people who want to know everything. If you feel like shit after the surgery or end up in the hospital getting a blood transfusion you will probably be reading this in the hospital bed saying, "that's what he was talking about". You may wanna at least skim it over or read the summary at the end. There are some good tips to share with your doctor in it on how to minimize blood loss (hopefully they already know this, but maybe not).

Hemoglobin is a protein molecule in red blood cells. Its function is to carry oxygen from the lungs to the body's tissues. After unloading the oxygen it carries carbon dioxide from the tissues back to the lungs. About 70% of the iron in our body is found in the red blood cell.

Your hemoglobin level is measured in a blood test known as a complete blood count (CBC). The hemoglobin level is expressed as the amount of hemoglobin in grams (gm) per deciliter (dL) of whole blood A deciliter is 100 milliliters. The normal ranges for hemoglobin depend on the age and, beginning in adolescence, the gender of the person.

Adult males: 14 to 18 gm/dL
Adult women: 12 to 16 gm/dL

Anemia

Anemia is known as the medical condition in which the red blood cell count of hemoglobin is less than normal. Essentially, **anemia** is a condition in which you don't have enough healthy red blood cells to carry adequate oxygen to the body's tissues.

The scope of this chapter is not to give you the information to self diagnosis yourself with anemia but to give you an overview of what your doctor is thinking and his or her concerns.

Once it is determined that your hemoglobin is below the normal, one looks at the MCV (mean corpuscular volume). This is the size of the red blood cell. It is a number that is in the same blood test report. If it is less than 81 we consider this microcytic anemia, if it is 81-100 is it considered normocytic anemia, and above 100 it is called macrocytic anemia. There are a host of other tests and parameters that are looked at to further diagnose the exact cause of the anemia, but it is important to understand that anemia is a symptom. Anemia is not a disease. It is important to find out what is causing the anemia.

The most common cause of anemia is iron deficiency anemia. This is a microcytic anemia. Anemia from blood loss is a normocytic anemia. B12, folate deficiency, alcoholism, and many medications cause macrocytic anemia.

As a general rule in my office, we do not perform liposuction on anyone with a hemoglobin less than 12 gm/dl. This number will drop, oftentimes fairly dramatically following liposuction. As described above, the hemoglobin level is expressed in a ratio 12 grams / 1 deciliter of blood. As with any ratio, this number can be lowered by decreasing the top number (numerator) or increasing the bottom number (denominator). So what happens after surgery??

First lets understand some of the 'juices' of the body: The **interstitial fluid i**s defined by the National Cancer Institute as:

Fluid found in the spaces around cells. It comes from substances that leak out of blood capillaries (the smallest type of blood vessel). It helps bring oxygen and nutrients to cells and to remove waste products from them. As new interstitial fluid is made, it replaces older fluid, which drains towards lymph vessels. **When it enters the lymph vessels, it is called lymph.** Also called tissue fluid.

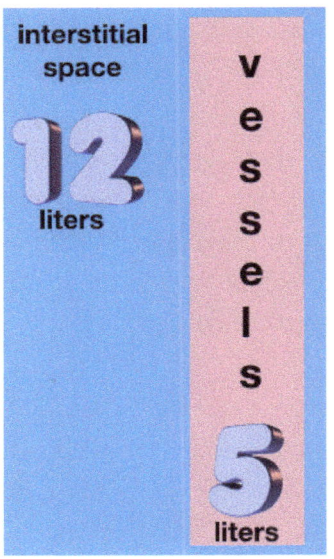

The normal amount of interstitial fluid in the body is

12 liters.
The normal amount of blood in the blood vessels is 5 liters.

The surgery starts and fluid is injected into the tissue before liposuction. We refer to this as tumescent fluid. This fluid adds to the amount of interstitial fluid.

Intravenous fluid is given by anesthesia (IV fluid). Although it is placed into a vein and is supposed to stay there, because liposuction has started, the blood vessels become very leaky. This allow for the healing cells of the body to exit the blood vessels, and go the areas of injury. This iv fluid leaks out and adds to the interstitial fluid.

Liposuction continues and removes a small portion of interstitial fluid. More bleeding from injury continues and the blood leaves vessels and goes to the interstitial space. Most of the bleeding from lipo goes to the interstitial space and not out of the body.

To make up for the perceived blood loss and lower blood pressure, anesthesia will often give more fluid which will cause a relative anemia (since its demonstrated as a percent). All of these things will lower the hemoglobin and hematocrit.

After surgery, the fluid in the interstitial space will slowly start to enter the blood stream. This too will account for a lower hemoglobin and hematocrit.

From the anesthesia the blood pressure will often be low after surgery. Many anesthesia providers without a good understanding of the liposuction will often look at the canister of fat/fluid removed and give more intravenous fluid than necessary. This is counter productive not only lowering the hemoglobin level but creating a massive amount of swelling that could take weeks for the patient to get relief from.

$$\frac{\text{Blood loss during surgery (↓'s the number)}}{\uparrow \text{ iv fluids given during surgery/recovery} \atop \uparrow \text{ fluid injected into tissue from tumescent that is absorbed}} = \downarrow \text{ hemoglobin}$$

We have seen the hemoglobin drop as many points as 4 gm/dl from its starting point. Before surgery we require all of our patients to undergo medical clearance by their primary care physician to make sure they can tolerate this drop. With or without liposuction, 5 L of tumescent solution decreases the hematocrit by 10%

We additionally try to educate our patients about how they will feel after surgery, how they will look, and how much leaking is expected from the liposuction openings made during the recovery process. We have had patients panic and end of up in the emergency room. An emergency room provider, not likely familiar with liposuction, will take a CBC and see a low hemoglobin and a stable patient and decide to transfuse a patient with blood. This is something we try to avoid not only because is it an added expense, wasteful of resources, inconvenient, and a transfusion is not without risk.

An anemic patient will be weak and dizzy. The patient may have some shortness of breath and a rapid heartbeat. Difficulty sleeping, headache, and leg cramps are not uncommon. The lips of our patients are typically pale in color as are the conjunctiva of the eyes. Patients may have cravings for chewing ice, a phenomenon known as pica.

That being said, there are some serious problems that are consistent with these symptoms. If you are experiencing these things, you should notify your doctor immediately and let them assess if it is serious or not. Do not trust your friend who used to date a doctor from Dominican Republic or anyone with a Google medical degree.

Aside from making sure our patients are healthy enough to tolerate a hemoglobin drop, we require our patients to stay overnight in a local accommodation we help set up. On post operative day 1 we send a nurse to check on the patient, assess the patient, photos are sent to me (Dr B), and assuming everything looks normal the patient heads to their final recovery destination. Patients from other states or countries are required to stay 7-10 days.

Additionally, we purchased a machine often used in the hospital for orthopedic surgery, known as a cell saver. This machine accepts the blood that is aspirated during liposuction. It purifies the blood, removing any fat particles that may be in the blood and prepares it for transfusion. We then give the blood back to the patient. This is not a blood transfusion from another person. This is the patients blood that was lost during the surgery.

The best thing about giving blood back is it helps maintain the patient's hemoglobin level and keeps the blood pressure up without needing to over hydrate the patient with iv fluid. Generally anesthesia providers will use normal saline (0.9% Sodium Chloride) or Lactated Ringers as a fluid replacement surgery surgery. We call these fluids crystalloid fluids. They are isotonic with blood. However we need to give 3 liters of these fluids to get the same effect of 1 unit of packed red blood cells. Over hydrating the patients with too much intravenous fluid is harmful for wound healing and can cause prolonged swelling that can last for weeks.

Very few doctors have this machine. It is fairly expensive and the disposables for each case are expensive and one time use. I do believe if you do aggressive liposuction, this machine is very important to have in your office. As a patient I would ask my doctor about it as well. Low hemoglobin after surgery is probably the most common reason a person is admitted to a hospital after surgery. This machine can help prevent an unnecessary admission and a very dangerous situation. At the time that I write this, having this machine is not the standard of care. I do believe as more doctors are doing liposuction, as the procedures continues to be the fasted growing cosmetic procedure, and patients expectations of dramatic results continue to grow there will be more patients who get into trouble with a low hemoglobin after surgery. At some point legislation will likely catch up and having this machine will be the standard of care if you want to perform this surgery.

The other step that can be done to minimize blood loss is the use of transexemic acid (TXA). It has been used initially in oral and maxillofacial surgery and then trauma surgery and has been shown to decrease the amount of blood loss during liposuction. Ask your doctor about this as well. This is relatively new at the time this publication is being done but i am confident will be the standard of care in a few years. It makes a huge difference in decreasing the blood loss and has little to no risk. I use it in in the iv and in the fluid we use to to inject before removing the fat.

Epinephrine is routinely used in the numbing fluid to minimize bleeding and left to sit for 18 minutes before liposuction commences.

If you have a history of anemia or know your hemoglobin runs low, if is best to have it checked over a month before surgery. It takes time to get your hemoglobin level up. This is particularly true in those that have had massive weight loss surgery. Assuming the cause of the anemia is iron deficiency anemia which is the most common a simple answer is to take iron supplements. Iron supplements will constipate you, so it is best to take a time release iron supplement. Examples of such are SlowFe® or Ferrosequel™. This takes weeks to allow for the hemoglobin to creep up. Patients can get iron infusions that can help more quickly that must be coordinated by your physician. Epogen® or Procrit® can be injected to raise the levels up quickly, however this can be expensive. It takes some coordination and planning, but one could even donate a unit of their own blood weeks in advance of their surgery and have arrangements made to receive their own blood in a form of a transfusion after surgery. This is an added expense and does require a fair amount of leg work but getting your own blood back is better than getting an emergency allogeneic (donor) blood transfusion in the hospital.

In summary hemoglobin levels are of critical importance before and after surgery. After aggressive liposuction one should expect a drop in hemoglobin that a person should be healthy enough to tolerate and the hemoglobin should be high enough to tolerate a significant dip. Our rule of thumb is a hemoglobin of 12 or greater is safest. A cell saver is an important machine that can make the recovery much easier and safer for a patient. One unit of packed red blood cells can raise the hemoglobin 3 points. If at all possible it is best to have your blood hemoglobin checked before your menstrual cycle and to schedule the surgery before your menstrual cycle. If you do get your period the day of surgery, that is not an absolute contraindication for surgery but it is a good idea to tell your surgeon beforehand, but I am hoping they will notice.

Chapter 20: What is the deal with these embolisms?

"Man is as old as his arteries."
Dr. Thomas Sydenham

Before getting too ahead of ourselves I wanted to give some basic explanations to clarify some words.

Blood clots are globs of blood that at one time was liquid but now became solid.

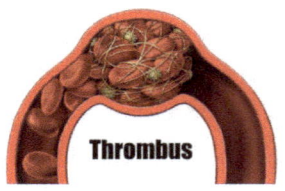

When this process happens inside of a blood vessel, this glob is called a thrombus.

A thrombus that dislodges from its place and travels down a vessel is called an embolus.

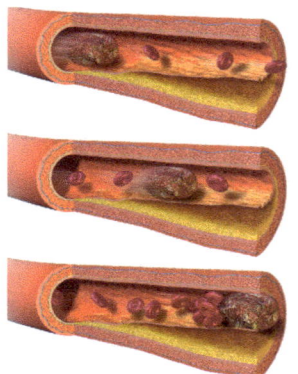

If that emboli gets stuck downstream because it is too large to pass in the vessel, and blocks blood flow around it is called an embolism.

A Pulmonary embolism (PE) is when a clot breaks loose from a distant site and lodges itself in the small vessels that supply blood to the lungs. The common source of these clots is in the legs and they are known as deep vein thrombosis (DVT).

A PE can be life threatening or can lead to permanent damage. The symptoms depend on the size of of the emboli, the health of the person, if there is more than one, and what it is occluding. Half of the people with PEs have no symptoms while others can have:
1. shortness of breath,
2. chest pain, worse with deep inspiration
3. rapid heart rate
4. dizziness or lightheadedness
5. cough (productive that may have blood in it)

These symptoms are quite scary in that in some degree, they are symptoms that are consistent with any surgery of this nature. It is very easy for a patient to have these symptoms after and the patient and even the doctor attributes these complaints to the surgery, and misses the diagnosis of a PE. A pulmonary embolism should always be considered when these symptoms present themselves.

If a PE is suspected, the next step is to go to the emergency room for the proper diagnostic workup. A diagnosis of PE cannot be made based solely on clinical examination or on the phone.

A PE can happen in the general population without surgery but is more common:
- after surgery
- Cancer

- A personal or family history of venous blood clots or pulmonary embolisms
- Heart disease
- Broken hip, leg or other trauma
- Inactivity: e.g. due to surgery, injury, bedrest, prolonged sitting (long car trips or flights), or paralysis
- Smoking
- Certain medications such as birth control pills, hormone replacement therapy, or Tamoxifen
- Pregnancy and childbirth
- Advanced age
- Obesity

An embolism does not have to be from a blood clot. During a fat transfer (BBL), fat can enter the circulation by injecting in the incorrect area causing a fat embolism. A fat embolism almost always presents itself on the operating room table. If it does occur in the operating room, there is no predictable, reversible treatment for this. Life supporting measures are taken (Advanced Cardiac Life Support) and Emergency Services are activated but usually the outcome is fatal. I am not trying to scare you out of doing the procedure, just trying to educate you so you chose a well qualified doctor and make an informed decision. When done correctly, the risk of this complication is almost 0.

Why is this surgery more of a risk in creating fat embolisms?

The layers of the butt that we are now discussing, going from superficial to deep is
- skin
- fat
  - superficial fat

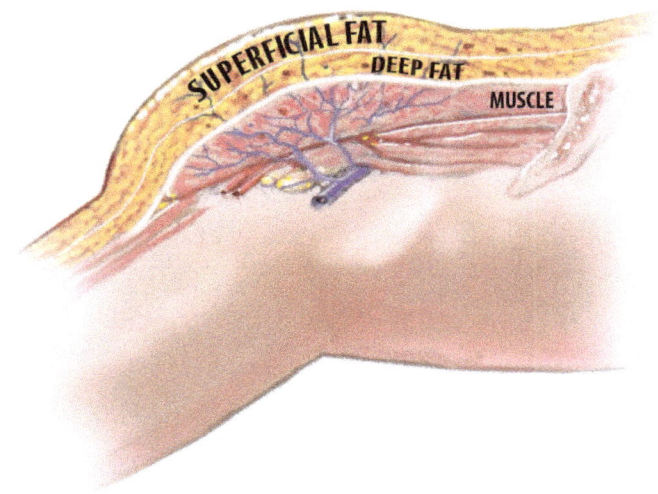

- Scarpa's fascia (a thin layer of tissue that separates the superficial and deep portions of fat-white line on the diagram)
- deep fat
- fascia (white line between the yellow and pink) covering the muscle
- gluteus maximus muscle
- deep vessels

The fascia overlying the muscle is quite strong and is excellent seal to separate the muscle from the fat. **There is no fascia on the the underside of the muscle.** Surgeons did an experiment on a cadaver. They used apple sauce that was made to be the same consistency as fat. They injected it in the top part inside of the muscle. As time passed, it was found to be at the deepest part of the muscle where the blood vessels reside.

2 things have to happen to get a fat embolism.
1. Fat needs to be introduced in or around the large vessels deep beneath the muscle

2. There has to be a break or tear in the veins to allow for the fat to enter the blood stream.

When examining the autopsy reports of the BBL deaths in Florida, all the victims had blood in and/or around the vessels, even though the surgeons denied injecting the fat into or through the muscle.

After these 2 things happens, the fat enters the blood stream and acts as a mechanical plug preventing blood blood downstream to where it clogs. In the heart, lung, or brain. If large enough will cause distress followed by almost immediate death.

The two proposed theories of how the fat enter the bloodstream are:
1. **Direct injection** into the vessels, deep into the muscle. For this to occur, the surgeon must be pretty far off in their control of the cannula tip, unless there is a very poor understanding of the anatomy. Additionally to actually get the cannula into the vessel (especially a large blunt cannula) is very difficult to do. Researchers actually tried to do it on cadavers and had a hard time doing so. (true, this were not live patients and the tissues may not be as welcoming as a live person)
2. **Indirect injection** around a torn vessel. This is the more likely occurrence. Once a cannula is inserted below the fascia the fascia works as an excellent seal trapping the fat in the muscle and there is a negative pressure in the vein that almost works like a vacuum that sucks the fat up. The fat

follows the path of least resistance and enter the blood stream.

The tear in the vein can result from:
1. trauma by a cannula
2. or even stretching the tissue It has been shown that manipulating the tissue even a few millimeters can create a sheering tear in this sized vein

This vein is quite large, has no valves at this point and is located near much larger tributary vessels. And again, there is no fasciae below the muscle to protect the muscle from the vessels.

If fat does enter the blood stream there are no protocols to treat this problem specifically. The closest model of treatment is the treatment for pulmonary embolism from a blood clot. The difference is the blood clot can be dissolved while fat causing an occlusion cannot.

Studies looking at the time of death after the fat embolism has shown it to be quickly after occurrence. 8 of 13 (61.1%) deaths in Mexico occurred during surgery. 77.7% deaths in Colombia occurred during surgery. In the US 8 of 10 reported fat embolism deaths that occurred demonstrated symptoms within minutes or hours of the surgery.

Extracorporeal Membrane Oxygenation (ECMO) can be a life saving procedure for pulmonary embolism and is performed in some hospitals. There are no reported cases of using ECMO to treat fat embolism originating from a fat transfer. This machine allows for oxygenation of the blood and bypasses the lung and heart. Not all hospitals have it, and even if they did, these fat transfers are typically performed in the surgeon's office not a hospital.

While prevention is clearly the most important part of dealing with a fat embolism, protocols for the treatment of such occurrences continue to be discussed. ECMO is in the conversation for the treatment of the macro fat embolism.

Chapter 21: Is it Safe?

"The most important person in the operating room is the patient."
                                    Dr. Russell John Howard

(This chapter gets a little serious and technically detailed (sorry), but I believe it is necessary to answer this question appropriately, and risking your life for an elective procedure deserves this detail)

1 in 3,000 people who get a BBL are going to die on the table???????

That is what the media is running in so many stories as a panicked craze spreads across the cosmetic surgery community.

Where do this come from?

It started here:

in 2015 a survey was performed by the Mexican Association of Reconstructive, Plastic and Aesthetic Surgery showing 22 deaths from fat transfer to the butt. Upon autopsy damage was shown in the gluteal vessels along with fat in the deep muscle. Their recommendations from the study was that this procedure should be done carefully and injections into the <u>deep</u> muscle should be avoided.

The Multi-Society Task Force for Safety in Gluteal Fat Grafting (ASAPS, ASPS, ISAPS, IFATS, ISPRES), representing board-certified plastic surgeons around the world, recently released a practice advisory (2017). I am sure with the best intentions, their findings were quite alarming.

They showed an unusually high mortality rate (death rate) from this cosmetic procedure to be estimated to be as high as 1:3000, greater than any other cosmetic surgery

This sounded the alarm all over the news! The UK essentially banned the BBL from being performed. in 2018 the British Association of Aesthetic Plastic Surgeons asked its members to stop performing the operation until more studies were done. There was fear Florida would put legislation forward banning it as well, just as they banned liposuction a few years back (later reversing their decision). Instead, Florida made it ILLEGAL for a doctor to inject fat into the muscle during a BBL. Many doctors, some "high profile" doctors on television are coming out saying this surgery should be banned. They goofy.

The chance of a woman dying during delivering a child is 0.3:1,000. Should we stop women from having babies? The odds of dying in a car crash is 1:77. Should we all not leave the house? This is a public health problem that requires experienced doctors to educate the less experienced doctors and the public. I don't care if you are Board certified plastic surgeon with 10,000 various surgeries under your belt, chances are, you didn't learn this surgery during residency. It has become most popular over the past few years, and most doctors after reading or going to a CE lecture learn by doing their first one. On a patient. In their office.

Patients will continue to enhance their butt, even by making bad decisions. Plump parties in hotels of peoples homes are reported all the time on the news. Some may go to unsafe countries where the death rate is even higher. We owe it to our patients to be trained properly and deliver this great surgery in a safe manner.

Before you read this chapter I recommend you first read the chapter that explains what a fat embolism is. This is super important and I want to make sure you guys are fully educated on this.

This is what everyone is talking about.

The cause of mortality is uniformly fatal **fat embolism** due to fat entering the venous circulation associated with injury to the gluteal veins. In every patient who has died, at autopsy, fat was seen within the gluteal muscle. In no case of death has fat been found only in the subcutaneous plane.

Here is a closer look at the medical literature.

Here are the *Recommendations from the ASERF Task Force on Gluteal Fat Grafting* in **bold**:

1. **Avoid injecting into the deep muscle.**

    This is not good advice. The muscle should be completely avoided. The muscle is covered in a layer called the fascia. As long as the fascia is not violated and the fat is injected above it (and therefore not in the muscle) there is no chance of getting a fat embolism.

2. **Use ≥4.1 mm diameter single hole injection cannula.**

    This is true. I personally use a 5 mm cannula, A smaller cannula is more likely to bend in the butt and you could loose your whereabouts and enter the muscle by mistake. Additionally a smaller cannula can more easily penetrate the muscle and enter a vessel.

3. **Avoid downward angulation of the cannula.**

    Yes, to avoid the muscle.

4. **Position patient and place incisions to create a path that will avoid deep muscle injections.**

    Yes. Some people say a jack knife position of the table is more dangerous. I feel comfortable with it, but for those less experienced I would agree with this.

5. **Maintain constant 3-dimensional awareness of the cannula tip.**

    Yup.

6. Only inject when cannula is in motion.
This is true however I would also say to inject only while withdrawing One can insert the cannula in the wrong place but are less likely to cause a problem if they haven't injected yet. It is safer to insert the cannula to verify the endpoint, then inject as you withdraw, One's withdrawal game should be strong.

7. Consider pulmonary fat embolism in unstable intra- and postoperative patients.
Always!

8. Review gluteal vascular anatomy.
Absolutely. How can you drive somewhere if you don't know the roads to get there.

9. Include the risk of fat embolism and surgical alternatives in the informed consent process.
You, the patients should totally understand the risks you are about to take. Now ya know.

They reported 1:3,000 BBL report in a death! Is 1 in 3,000 BBLs an accurate reflection of what is going on out there???
NO WAY! The study was heavily scrutinized by many surgeons and much of the forthcoming information was found in Dr. Delvecchio's article in response to the study)

Here are some problems with the study that done :

WHY THE NUMBERS ARE PROBABLY OFF:
1. This was an anonymous web-based survey that was sent to 4843 plastic surgeons worldwide, only 692 surgeons replied. They reported 198,857 cases of fat grafting into the butt. They reported 32 fatalities from pulmonary fat emboli as well as 103 nonfatal pulmonary fat emboli. The response rate of this survey was 14%. Then there are a large population of cosmetic surgeons doing BBLs that are not plastic surgeons and did not participate in the study. Many large BBL practices like Dr. Miami and myself were never asked to participate (probably close to 2,000 BBLs performed last year by the two of us alone without a fat embolism)

2. Even those who *did* respond, were anonymous so maybe they replied more than once. Admitted by the authors, there was no measures to prevent this.

3. There is something called *recall bias*: it is when the person cannot recall all the details of their cases.

4. There is something called *participation bias:* it is when the surgeons who had a death were more likely to respond to do a service to the community or because of guilt while those without a death may be more likely to simply ignore the invitation to do the

survey. Or are they *less* likely to participate because of shame.

5. There is something called *subject bias:* it is when a participant acts in a way that they think the examiner wants them to act when they think they know the reason for the survey. The incidence of deaths and the total amount of surgeries performed may not be accurate.

6. Other issues with this US study included:

- there was no consideration of fat particle size

- patient position during injection was not mentioned (flat, on side, table bent in a jack knife position)

- harvest technique? (size of cannula, power assisted, waterjet, vaser, laser, manual)

- injection technique used? (power injected versus by hand)

- how large were the syringes used for injection?

- where did the venous injury occur

- did they inject in the plane they thought they did

- how much fat was injected?

- Surgeons were asked to report the planes in which they "typically" inject but were not asked what they did in the specific instances of each death

- there is no actual delineation between superficial and deep muscle

- preparation technique

- incision location

Some of thee important factors are discussed below from other studies and personal beliefs.

A much better designed study was performed in Brazil. A total of 853 of the 5655 Board-Certified Brazilian plastic surgeons answered the survey. The mortality (death) rate estimated was 1: 20,117 cases. And, by the way, 76% of these plastic surgeons learned about BBL in their residency. The conclusions made from this study was: a maximum of 500 ml per buttock subcutaneously (under the skin and above the muscle) only, via superior gluteal incisions (incision on the top of the butt), using 3 to 4 mm diameter cannulas for fat harvesting and injection, and keep the patients in observation for 23 hours. I agree with some of these points, but not all.

Therefore, stay mentally focused, alert, and aware of the cannula tip at every moment; be vigilant about following the intended trajectory with each stroke and feel the cannula tip through the skin. Consider positioning that can favor superficial approaches, such as table jackknife. Use cannulas that are resistant to bending during injection and recognize that Luer connectors can loosen and bend during surgery.

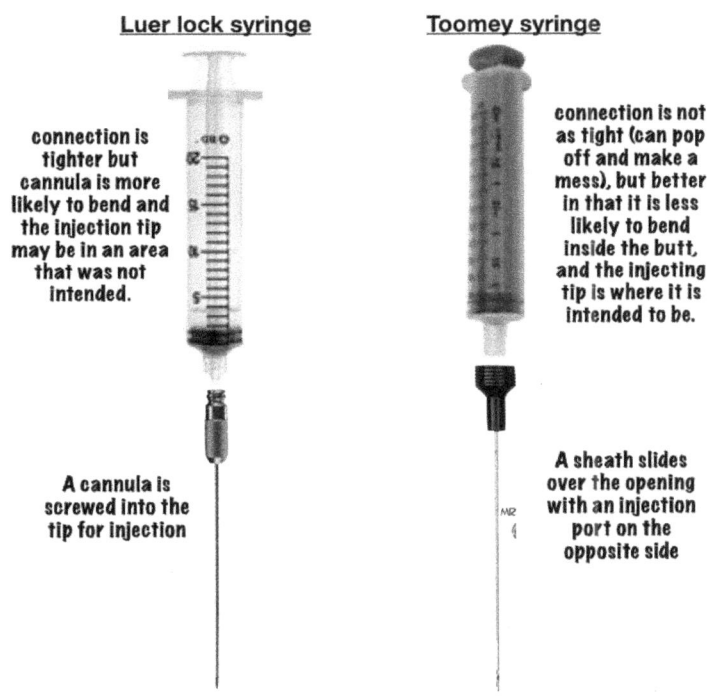

Luer lock syringe

connection is tighter but cannula is more likely to bend and the injection tip may be in an area that was not intended.

A cannula is screwed into the tip for injection

Toomey syringe

connection is not as tight (can pop off and make a mess), but better in that it is less likely to bend inside the butt, and the injecting tip is where it is intended to be.

A sheath slides over the opening with an injection port on the opposite side

Although this study did not show that the amount of experience has any relevance in the safety, I would not agree with this. Here is a distribution of doctors that were surveyed in this study.

This is the number of BBL procedures done over the course of these doctors careers.

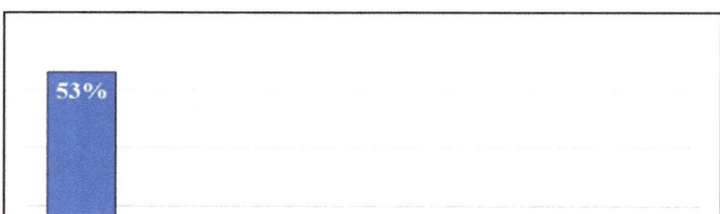

Table 4. General Characteristics of Microscopic Fat Embolism and Macroscopic Fat Embolism

	MIFE	MAFE
Causal agent	Microscopic fat generally in liquid form or micelles that can form microemboli	Macroscopic fat that groups into clots forming macroemboli
Pathophysiology	By effect of lipase, fatty acids are released from microemboli, producing alveolar and capillary irritation with hemodynamic alterations	Fat cells clot immediately obstructing the venous blood vessels and heart by a mechanical effect
Start	24–72 hr postoperatively	Immediate, intraoperative; from the beginning of surgery to 1–2 hr postoperatively
Clinical presentation	Gurd and Wilson criteria for fat embolism; effects on microcirculation; pulmonary, cutaneous, and central nervous system disorders	Similar to pulmonary thromboembolism; mechanical effect on the heart producing sudden cardiac failure
Diagnosis	Clinical; computed tomography (ground-glass opacity and pleural effusion)	Clinical; sudden onset, which begins when the fat is injected; cardiac failure
Prognosis	Mortality of 10–30%, depending on how fast the management starts	Based on published reports almost 99%
Treatment	Respiratory and hemodynamic support measures in the intensive care unit	Currently not described; aggressive cardiovascular support; mainly experimental (ciclesonide, rosuvastatin, percutaneous embolectomy)
Prevention	Avoid injecting liquid fat; adequate hydration; avoid injection in very vascularized areas	The most important factor is to avoid deep intramuscular injection into the medial portion of the gluteus

MIFE, microscopic fat embolism; MAFE, macroscopic fat embolism.

Speaking as a surgeon who has greatly surpassed 1000 cases in my career, I disagree that experience is a non factor in safety. A working knowledge of the anatomy, and the technique of injection is something that takes experience to master. I, as a patient, would not feel comfortable having someone who in their career has done less than 50 BBLs, not only because of the safety, but to master the aesthetic aspect of it takes experience. To further support my point there was a recent study in India looking at trends in plastic surgery. The surgeons who presented the fewest complications were those who operated on more than 70 cases per year. It is the consensus that surgeons more accustomed to performing these procedures have better knowledge of the safety limits of the procedure

In 2016, Conde-Green et al published a systemic review of the literature and meta-analysis, and found 19 articles made up of a total of 4105 patients. They found that 46.7% of the articles recommended fat injections into both the subcutaneous and intramuscular planes, 26.7% into only the intramuscular planes, and 26.7% into the subcutaneous or subfascial planes. This is frightening. Doctors who are not properly up to date with current research and training will kill more patients. The only acceptable safe plane to inject the fat in a BBL is the subcutaneous plane, above the muscle.

Other often cited studies include the aforementioned survey in Mexico and Colombia, where they examined deaths after injections of fat in the buttock. Interestingly, the amounts of fat infiltrated in the deaths were not large volumes, with the largest amount being 300 cc per buttock, with an average of 214 cc. Further supporting the main factor causing the problem is the muscle area where fat is injected not how much.

While other studies do not complete demonize muscular fat injections, they recommend not injecting into the part of the butt near the midline where the majority of the large vessels reside. Basically a zone 6-8 cm (2-3 inches) from the midline (butt crack).

Some articles recommend not injecting the top part of the fat that is collected. This refers to the fat canister after the fat is collected settles and separates itself. The top layer is oily and usually minimal. This is not recommended for re-injection. Making sure the patient is properly hydrated by anesthesia is important to help eliminate a small amount of free fatty acids that could enter the bloodstream potentially from this top layer

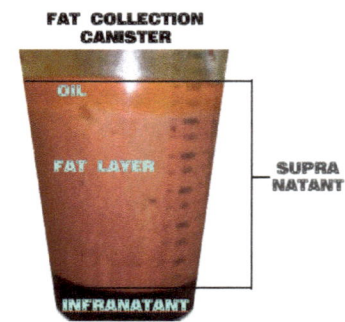

This point leads us to touch on the difference between microscopic fat embolism versus macroscopic fat embolism. Most of the concern and attention that we have focused on and what has become a major public health concern is the macroscopic fat embolism. Macroscopic fat embolism are totally attributable to a mechanical event and that the prognosis is very poor, because these types of problems are usually fatal. It is from injecting the fat layer into the muscles and therefore entering the deep vessels of the butt. A microscopic fat embolism is more likely to originate from the oily liquid layers of the collection canister. This chart summarize the difference between a microscopic and macroscopic fat embolism. It was taken from an article entitled, Critical Differences between Microscopic (MIFE) and Macroscopic (MAFE) Fat Embolism during Liposuction and Gluteal Lipoinjection, written by Lázaro Cárdenas-Camarena, M.D. Héctor Durán, M.D. José Antonio Robles-Cervantes, M.D., Ms.C., Ph.D. Jorge Enrique Bayter-Marin, M.D.

If depositing the fat into the correct location is the key element, obviously the angle of injections come into play. Studies looking at different incision entry points and angulations demonstrate the upper mid-gluteal port produced no neurovascular injury at angles of 0° and −10° but was found to produce complications at −30°.

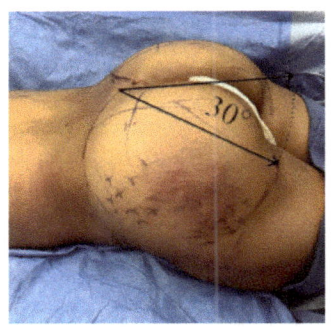

The upper midline incisions is believed to better protect an inadvertent dive

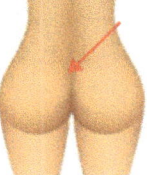

deep into the muscle as the sacrum bone prevents poor angulation. For a rookie injector this is probably a good idea, but with experience I do believe the lower incisions are safe and are often required to get the best cosmetic result.

In simple terms, if your surgeon accidentally injects fat into a large vein deep directly or by injecting in the muscle of your butt and having the fat migrate to the deep vessels the fat can enter your circulation. This fat can travel into your heart or lung. If this happens, depending on how severe the occlusion you can die instantaneously. There is no cure to reverse a fat embolism. A small one requires supportive measures and the body can break it down. A large fat embolism can result in instant death. For this reason, I would want to go to an expert.

Newer, better studies are now being published showing more realistic and optimistic numbers from this surgery now that surgeons are more aware of the risks and guidelines. In 2020, Dr. Luis Rios reported a mortality of 1:15,000 mortality for BBL after subcutaneous injections were made the standard of care. Hopefully this research will receive as much press as the one showing the extremely high death rate.

This surgery **is** a safe surgery when done correctly. Long before these guidelines were in place by this advisory counsel, I gave courses to doctors on how to do this correctly and safely. My advice was quite similar: large blunt cannulas for injection avoid piercing the veins, avoid deep injections, injecting the fat while the cannula is parallel to the table is a safe way to insure there is no accidental injection into the vessels.

The two ways to inject fat into the butt is by hand or by using a power injector. I do not think the results are very different between the two techniques. By hand the fat is transferred into 60 cc toomey syringes and injected using a 5 mm blunt cannula. The average positive pressure generated by such a syringe is 80" Hg. The HVP pump from Wells Johnson can create a pressure up to 40" Hg and allows you to set the upper limit so the machine automatically stops if more resistance is encountered.

I personally like the power injector better:
- It is a little faster
- Less surgeon fatigue
- It is a closed system (the fat goes from the body to the container back into the body), and less likely to be contaminated by handling.
- It is neater (the fat with the syringes gets very greasy and many times, I had pushed the syringe and the top flew off)
- It is pressure controlled to not allow fat to be injected too deep by modifying the pressure on the machine in addition to the flow rate.

The only true advantage for doing it by hand is you can theoretically pull back the syringe to make sure there is no blood in the syringe before injecting. This can confirm you are not in a vessel. However, if you are injecting in the level below the skin and over the muscle, there are no vessels that you should encounter. The theory of aspiration (pulling back the syringe to check if you are in vessel) sounds great, but in reality it is difficult to do so, the needle can still move while injecting, it is hard to see and you cannot fill the syringe fully if you need to leave some room to pull back. It is cheaper for the surgeon, needing less disposable supplies.

I do not think as a patient, you really should be too concerned with which technique your doctor uses.

Once you have the fat in a container, then what?

If you let the fat simply sit there in the canister, the major parts will separate based on the weight of the components. The bottom part is called the infranatant. It is made of liquid containing: blood, tumescent (numbing fluid injected before liposuction), and some stem cells. Above that is the fat. Within the fat are stem cells that cannot be seen without a microscope.

And the very top of the fat is a thin layer of oil. This is a result of ruptured or damaged fat cells releasing their contents. If the fat is suctioned out under very high power (for example greater than 25 psi), more fat can be damaged and this layer will be thicker. This wastes more fat that could have

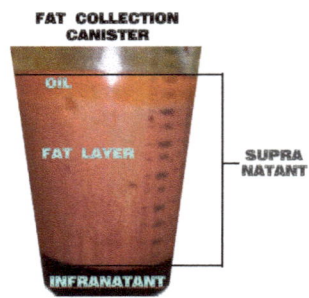

potentially been used for the transfer. Also, if the canister is not air tight, bubbles will fill the canister during the suctioning process. This will look like the little treasure chest with the bubbles in a fish tank, or like a little jacuzzi. This will also damage the fat and that oil layer will be larger.

Most doctors drain the bottom fluid and inject the fat. The fluid can be used in a device called a cell saver which extracts the red blood cells and allows for a transfusion of the blood you just lost. Not many offices have this device but it is so helpful to maintain your safety and we use it each week. If there is little fluid, it can be mixed with the fat (to maximize the stem cell population), or simply discarded in the biohazardous waste.

While injecting it is best to avoid injecting the oil layer. It can form a cyst in the body, and there is a risk of micro emboli as discussed above.

The only modification to the fat I do is to add antibiotics depending on the patients allergies. I use either Ancef, gentamicin or clindamycin or a combination depending on the patient. I give one standard dose per 1 liter of fat planned for injection.

Some people centrifuge the fat and spin it down, others don't. I personally do not. There has never been any science proving this to be beneficial. In fact, I think it may be detrimental to the fat. The way these fat transfers work, the fat itself works more like a scaffolding to hold the space in the butt for the stem cells to grow and take its place. Spinning the fat will damage the fat and further separate the stem cells from the fat. The stem cells will enter the liquid that will be discarded and the more of the fat cells will rupture from the spinning. This will be evident in an oil layer that will appear more on top top of the fat. This used to be more popular but very few do this anymore. Some physicians still do with their objective to leading you to believe their technique is special and better than the guy up the street. True story, admitted to me by a colleague. SMH

Does your doctor inject into the muscle or above the muscle?

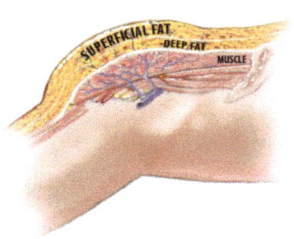

I know I am belaboring this point but it is so important. Again, here is the anatomy we are talking about.

Most well educated doctors now agree the safest place to put the fat is above the muscle and in the subcutaneous plane. When people hear about over the muscle, many automatically think about breast implants. Whether they should be placed above or below the muscle. In this situation there is no below the muscle it is above the muscle or *in* the muscle.

Because of the new guidelines, just about every doctor will say he or she injects above the muscle. The injections are historically done by feel, so whether it goes in the muscle cannot be confirmed. It is my belief that most doctors prior to the recent task force alarming report were injecting above the muscle and probably injecting a little (knowingly or unknowingly) into the muscle as well.

To further explain my point, when we get vaccines for example (tetanus shot), it is injected into the muscle. The length of the need used is 1.5 inches. That means when the needle is buried to the hub it is 1.5 inches into your butt. At this point you are universally considered to be in the muscle. That means the distance from the skin to the muscle in most people is less than 1.5 inches. I find it very hard to believe that we can inject 2,500 cc of fat into that small space blindly. We were probably injecting fat into the muscle without even knowing it, myself included.

My technique now has evolved to using an ultrasound device. This has opened up my eyes so much to get a look under the skin. You wouldn't fly a plane blindfolded would you? Using ultrasound will be more throughly explained in another chapter but it allows for SAFE injection above the muscle. You can scan the butt and see the areas that have room for more fat without risking a fat embolism. There is a thin layer (about 1 cm) that exists between the skin and fascia that can be injected to get a dent out. The cannula we use to inject is 5 mm (0.5 cm) in size. It would be very difficult to fit the cannula in this plane blindly without the help of an ultrasound unit. This should be and will be the standard of care eventually. Since using it, my results are better, I can better see problem areas and address them, and the results are safe. Me and my patients can sleep better at night.

FAT SHOULD NEVER BE PLACED IN THE MUSCLE. FAT SHOULD ONLY BE PLACED IN THE SUBCUTANEOUS TISSUE. If the desired outcome might require another procedure, then it's the doctors responsibility to manage the patient's expectations for multiple rounds of fat transfer. The concept of multiple rounds of grafting is very much accepted in hair transplants. Patients are well informed and ok with needing multiple rounds to get their desired results. This should be explained as well for patients undergoing a BBL if they want more extreme results. This is a safe procedure if done correctly by a skilled surgeon with experience in this particular procedure.

Chapter 22: Ultrasound assisted BBL (the safest way to do a BBL -in my opinion)

"The most important result of any surgical operation is a live patient."

Dr. Charles H. Mayo

Ultrasound assisted BBL- the only way this procedure is performed by me.

An ultrasound is a medical device that uses high-frequency sound waves to create an image. This is commonly used in pregnant women to check on the growing fetus, however it could create an image to see a person's abdominal and pelvic organs, muscles and tendons, or their heart and blood vessels. Some of the great attributes of an ultrasound is, it is a 'live feed' of what is happening, opposed to a still image. Another advantage of an ultrasound, is that it produces no radiation. Its mechanism is purely inaudible sound waves.

In my opinion there is no safer way to perform a BBL than with ultrasound. I call my machine our Rump Radar™.

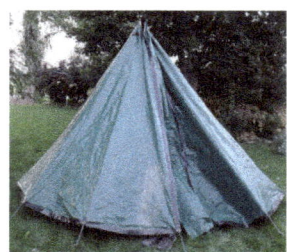
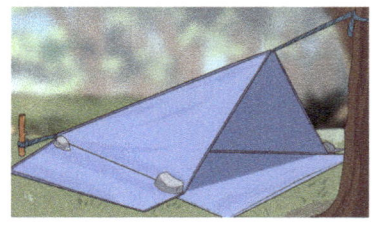

While injecting that fat, you can visualize where the cannula is at all times and watch the fat flow into the butt insuring it does not violate the muscle. Not only is it safer but the results that can be obtained are better.

There are some butts with some tight deformities that are hard to release and get fat to fit in. With ultrasound, you can properly visualize under the skin to see where andwhy is it is being held up to allow a better chance at correcting the problem. Even in the general shaping of the butt it is helpful.

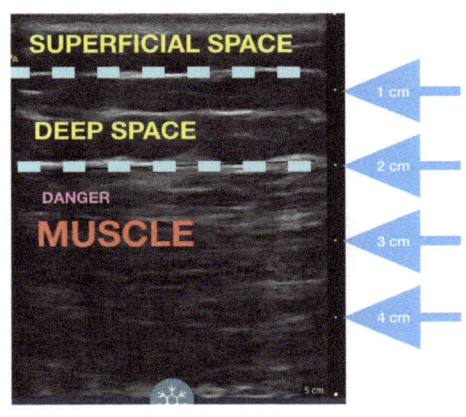

This is an ultrasound image of the butt before injection of fat. Please note how little the room is in the safe areas for fat injection. And again, the superficial space that would be injected to correct a dent is less than 1 cm. It was be very difficult to navigate a cannula 0.5 cm in diameter into this space without guidance.

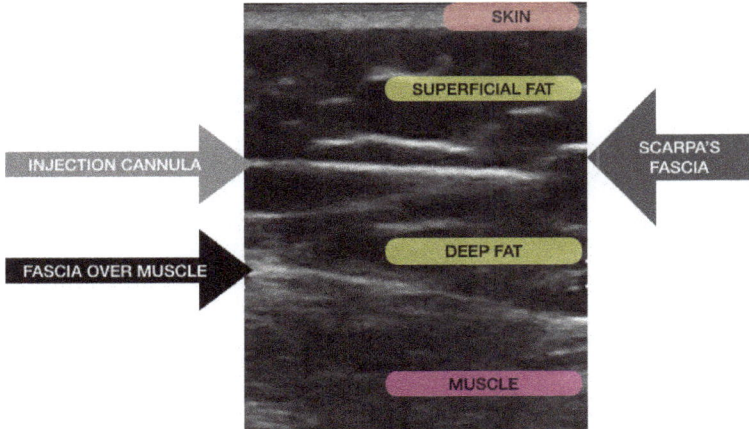

With the ultrasound, one can clearly see the delineation between the superficial and deep fat, separated by Scarpa's Fasica (see image below). To create a general bulking of the butt, I inject the fat under Scarpas's fascia but above the muscle. If someone has a dent or missing some superficial contouring, one would inject above Scarpa's fascia. This superficial space between the skin and Scarpa's is often 1 cm or less in size. The cannula we use is greater than 4 mm. It is challenging to fit the cannula in this space without seeing you are in it with an ultrasound. The space can even become smaller after injecting the fat in the deep fat layer which would compress the superficial space more.

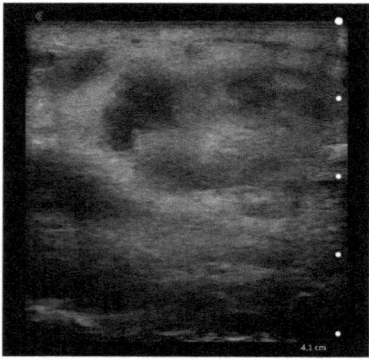

As the fat is injected, you can watch a cloud on the ultrasound image being created. This space is expanded due to the fat pushing the skin up.

Imagine the skin of the butt to be like a tent that needs to be put up. Once you put that peak of the tent up, the other areas become tighter and it is impossible to lift any of the other areas higher than than peak.

It is for that reason, I first lay down a nice foundation in the deep fat using the ultrasound. Then I go to the areas that require the most 'pop' (whether it be the hips or the projection back). The rest of the fat is trickled in to make everything flow smoothly.

Performing ultrasound during a BBL has no down side. It is my prediction that within time, this will be the standard of care. It does take more time, training, and some added expense for materials but a small price to pay to pretty much guarantee not injecting fat into a deep gluteal vessel and saving a patients' life.

Chapter 23: My recipe for a successful and safe technique

"I got beans, greens, potatoes, tomatoes, lamb, rams, hogs, dogs, beans, greens, potatoes, tomatoes, chicken, turkeys, rabbit. You name it!"

Shirley Ceasar

This is the safest way to inject fat into the butt, to get good results and not kill anyone.

This is only way I inject fat.

1. **Inject only in the subcutaneous level.** This is under the skin and above the muscle.
There is no superficial muscle
There should be no injecting into the muscle or under the fascia.

How do you know you never inject into the muscle? By ….

2. Inject using ultrasound. While injecting the fat you can see exactly where it is in real time. You first position your cannula in the right spot under direct visualization, then you inject.

3. Inject while withdrawing. While withdrawal is not always the preferred method in all of our activities (inappropriate reference intentional), it is the only way to inject fat. Leaving the fat cannula in one spot while injecting will create a lump of dead fat and injecting while moving forward or back and forth can create an unintentional path. Even if fat was not injected into this path, enough pressure can be created by adding a lot of fat in the subcutaneous plane to force and propel the fat down this path potentially into the muscle and headed for danger.

4. Use large rigid blunt single holed cannulas. The large blunt cannulas are less likely to penetrate into an erroneous path. Cannulas that are not rigid can bend inside the butt. They can appear they are in the right spot from the outside but can be too deep.

5. Be aware of the position of the butt in relation to the table and floor to try to inject parallel to the floor or upward, not downward. I use whatever incision I need to accomplish my cosmetic goal but making sure I am always aware of where my cannula tip is and I am injecting fat in a safe spot.

6. **The amount doesn't matter.** The amount of fat injected in the subcutaneous plane in my opinion does not put a patient more at risk of a fat embolism. I put in whatever looks good, and whatever the skin will allow to fit.

7. **Don't be a hero.** If there is a spot that is not responding well to expansion try your best but the enemy of good is better. By trying to push the envelope you can make things much worse.

8. Give realistic expectations. Explain to the patients beforehand potential limitations and expectations of their result. If you tell a patient before surgery it is an explanation, after surgery it becomes an excuse.

9. Use closed system power injector. Although the syringe method using a toomey syringe is ok, i do believe it increases the chance of an infection happening. It becomes quite messy and if you push the syringe too hard the cannula disconnects and the fat becomes wasted. Additionally it is very difficult to hold the syringe and cannula together while injecting and the ultrasound at the same time.

10. Add antibiotics to the fat. Depending on the patients allergies I always add any combination of gentamycin, bactrim, ancef, and/or clindaymcin to each canister of fat.

11. Take a picture of the fat collected. I always take a picture and put it in the patients chart. Sometimes people don't have enough fat for the results they want and this way they see how much was removed and injected. Other times we reach the legal and safe limit of fat removal (5 liters) and I can show them that this was achieved.

Chapter 24: Complications

"Show me a surgeon without complications, and I'll show you a surgeon who does not operate"
unknown

If you operate, you will have complications. There are too many variables involved that cannot be controlled otherwise. We are living biological creatures all with different bodies. If a surgeon said he has never had a complication, RUN!

In this chapter I will be discussing the more common complications and unfavorable outcomes.

We are discussing complications essentially for two different procedures: liposuction and fat injection. Although there are some complications that can happen in both facets of the procedures I have lumped them together as one procedure in this section.

With any surgery there are risks. This surgery is no different. The hot topic right now is the safety of the BBL referring to fat embolisms leading to death. This topic is deserving of its own focus therefore I have dedicated several chapters on that topic not covered here.

Things like pain, swelling, and bruising are consistent with any surgical procedure and these things typically resolve with time. These complaints usually escalate over the first 3 days and then slowly improve daily, until they fade away.

1. Swelling is a normal response to the surgical trauma of liposuction. Although the access holes for liposuction are few and small in size, the injury to the body is quite significant and far reaching. Swelling is to be expected. This is typically controlled with a post operative garment. The swelling is most noticeable around day 3 after surgery. As the infiltrated fluid, serum and broken down fat are absorbed by the body, the swelling changes to a more firm to woody consistency with no or minimal pain and discomfort by the end of 2-3 weeks. Yes, the majority of fat is removed with the liposuction cannula however there is fat that remains in the areas that was damaged by the cannula and wasn't removed. The body breaks this down over the next few weeks. By the end of 4 weeks, the majority of operated swollen areas start to soften in patches until the entire area shows a consistent softening by the end of 6-8 weeks. Lymphatic massages during this period help speed up and improve this process. Depending on the person, a normal soft feel could return as long as 3 months after the procedure.

Areas that are gravity dependent typically hold on to swelling longer than others. These areas include the legs and calves, the lower abdomen, and FUPA (mons area). These areas can take 6 months or even longer to resolve.

2. Bruising (ecchymosis) also will occur in all liposuction patients immediately after the procedure. This peaks by the end of 7-10 days, but generally disappears by 2-4 weeks after surgery. Unusually severe and persistent bruising/ecchymosis may be related to chronic smoking, use

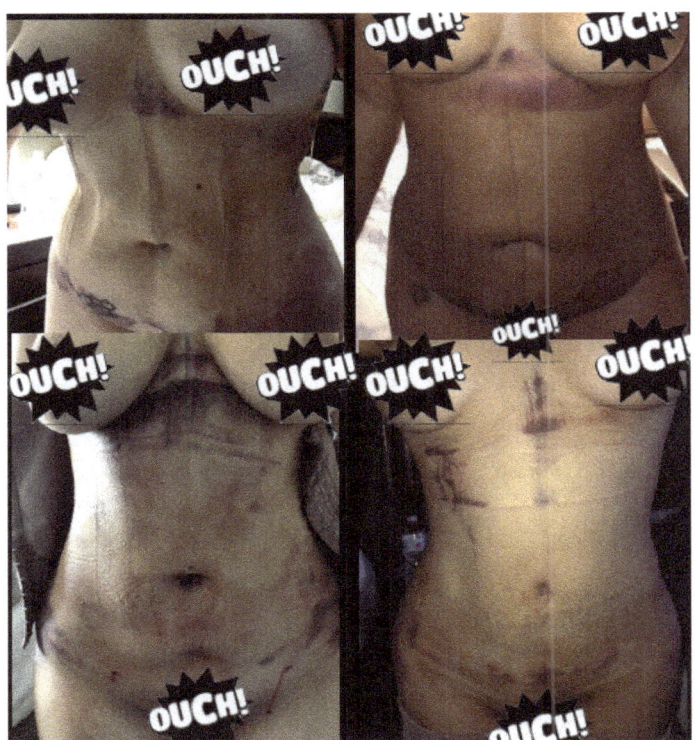

of blood thinners and abnormal bleeding/clotting profile. Here are some pictures of bruising that are normal within the first few days after surgery.

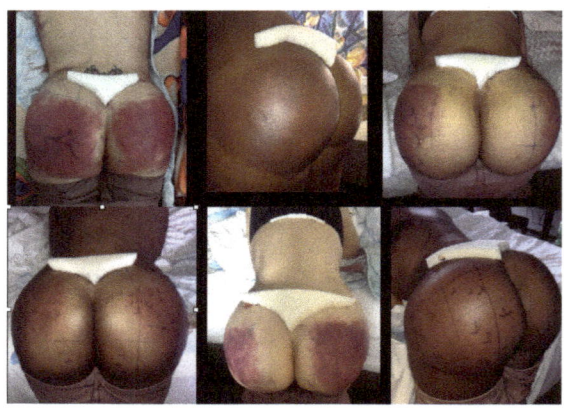

3. Seromas: A seroma is a collection of serous fluid. This fluid is composed of blood plasma that has seeped out of ruptured small blood vessels and inflammatory fluid produced by the injured and dying cells. Seromas are different from hematomas, which contain red blood cells, and different from abscesses, which contain pus and result from an infection. Serous fluid is also different from lymph. It may occur in a liposuctioned area due to tissue trauma, causing

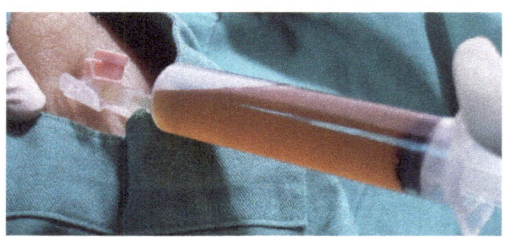

the destruction of the fibrous tissue network under the skin leading to a single cavity formation. It may also be due to significant damage to the lymphatics. For those that have had surgery in theses areas before they are more at risk of developing a seroma. If you had a seroma before, you are more at risk of getting another one. It has been shown to be more prevalent in ultrasound assisted liposuction (for example Vaser liposuction). Anecdotally, if a person is not wearing a proper fitting garment or the patient is taking it off too much or doing too much activity too early this too may contribute to a seroma formation. Those who have a lot of loose skin may be at an increased risk. If you can pull the skin away from the body more than 1.5 inches, a seroma is likely. A drain may be considered by your doctor.

Seromas usually present themselves around post operative day 7. The treatment is a simple sterile aspiration followed by proper compression. Sometimes this may require putting some extra foam padding in the areas where the seroma existed. This is most commonly found in the lower abdomen. Tapping on the area and watching a wave, is an indication of a seroma. Similar to throwing a stone in a pond, and watching the ripple. It has a similar appearance.

If a large amount of fluid is aspirated at the time of drainage the likelihood of it filling up again and recurring is high. For example draining more than 80 cc will likely require another drainage a few days later of usually less (perhaps 50 cc) until this number is essentially zero. There are situations where consistently, the amount drained keeps recurring. In those people often a drain is placed until that amount is essentially zero. A small seroma will be absorbed by the body. There are other options for chromic seromas that do not respond to serial aspirations. Your doctor may inject air into the tissue or inject tetracycline or triamcinolone into the seroma cavity to cause the cavity to get 'sticky'. After compression, it is one's hope the seroma cavity will collapse on itself, stick down, and not redevelop.

4. Infections can be serious but are not usually very common. During liposuction, they are quite uncommon. Some of this is due to the fact that lidocaine (the numbing agent) is bacteriostatic. The fat injection portion of the BBL is more likely but still uncommonly can get infected. These usually present as a warm area that could be different in color. If an infection presents, it will almost always present after the first week. The blood supply in the fatty layer of the butt is so poor that an infection, if ignored can become quite serious. If you believe you have developed an infection, inform your doctor right away, and you should be followed at least twice a week, depending on the severity. Whenever possible, it is best to treat the infection with antibiotics only. Ciprofloxacin, Levaquin, Bactrim, or Clindamycin have all been used to treat these infections with success.
 There are 3 stages of any infection.

1. Inoculum, is the first stage and usually is without clinical signs or symptoms. This is when the bacteria are growing in the wound.
2. Cellulitis is when the infection is spread diffusely in the tissue. The butt will appear red and tight. It is warm and often tender to touch. There can sometimes be fevers and or chills with this stage.
3. Abscess is the final stage of an infection. It is when the cellulitis stage matures and the infection collects in the form of a central area of pus. Pus is made up of dead white blood cells.

An abscess should be drained. Antibiotics travel in the blood stream and the blood supply to the abscess center is not very good. Therefore the antibiotics are not carried to the middle of the pus very well. Clindamycin is an antibiotic that has the best penetrance into an abscess cavity and it is only 33%. Many infections are a mixture of cellulitis and abscess. When the doctor feels over the cellulitis area if there is a small bouncy area, this is the opening to an abscess cavity and the spot where it needs to be drained. If pus is removed it is best to send it for a culture and sensitivity to see what bacteria caused the infection and what antibiotics it is sensitive and resistant to. If you are on antibiotics prior to the drainage, it can give a false culture but still antibiotics should be started as soon as possible. There are opportunist infections, where bacteria that did not cause the infection start to flourish. This is because the environment inside the wound had changed as a result of the causative infecting bacteria. Oftentimes the culture will grow a bacteria like Staph that got into the sample because it lives on the skin but has nothing to do with the cause of infection.

One should start with antibiotics as a first option and it should be sorted early. The problem with making a hole for drainage is fat added to the butt will take the path of least resistance. Usually the butt is filled with fat under a lot of pressure. If a hole is made in the butt to drain the infection, after the pus is expressed, fat can continuously drain from the hole. Particularly if the patient sits or even wears a tight garment, this pressure can cause the fat to be expressed from the hole. This can result in a cosmetic defect. However, if an abscess exists, again, it should be drained. The infection needs to be taken care of first. Leaving an infection to grow in an area with a poor blood supply can destroy all the fat. The cosmetic result can be addressed later.

If there is tight or indented area starting off in the butt, this area may require much manipulation to try to stretch it out during surgery. This can result in significant trauma to the butt (recipient) site. Rarely I have seen these spots develop 'granulomatous reactions' which look like infections but do not grow any bacteria. They can require a small incision to drain out the dead fat and they typically heal uneventfully. If ignored, they can rupture and then bacteria is introduced into the wound and can cause a secondary infection.

When a lot of trauma with the injection cannulas has occurred and the fat is injected more superficially than deep the blood supply to support the fat can be compromised. Sometimes small lesions that look like boils can occur that are often confused with infections. They too are granulomatous reactions to fat in a damaged recipient site. The treatment can vary from drainage, to steroids, to simply observation. A biopsy of the tissue is the best indicator of what it is.

5. A **hematoma** is a collection of blood under the skin in the skin where liposuction was performed. It is recommended that patients stop smoking and medications such as aspirin, clopidogrel, non-steroidal anti-inflammatory drugs, vitamin E, glucosamine, chondroitin, ginseng and ginkgo biloba at least 7 days before surgery to minimize their chance of getting a hematoma.

Small hematomas are generally left alone. Moderate sized hematomas should be allowed to liquefy and then aspirated followed by wearing proper compression garments. Large sized hematomas should be drained through the liposuction port or by repeat liposuctioning followed oftentimes by suction drains in selected cases.

6. Undercorrection is a complaint when fat is left behind after liposuction. Absolutely this can be the case. For the first few months however, this is often confused with swelling. This may also be confused with loose skin. When loose skin persists on the belly it appears wavy and it can appear as though there is irregular liposuction.

7. Overcorrection -The traditional way many of us were taught to do liposuction was to leave a protective layer of fat to prevent dents or contour irregularities. The desires of our patients have changed and in most of the younger patients we treat, this protective layer is suctioned as well. They want to be 'super snatched' and this is how it is done.

I still like to warn my patients on areas that are prone to look bad after an overcorrection. These areas include the inner thighs. This is most common areas for indentations as a result of thin skin is the inner thighs. I always demonstrate how thin the skin is on the inner thigh. Removing the fat here can leave a patient with 'crepey old lady skin'. If inner thigh lipo is to be performed, it should be conservative and deep. It should be done do create some space between the legs. The correction is doing a thigh lift, a skin tightening treatment like j plasma, or adding fat back to the area.

Another common area to create a dent is the outer aspect of the thighs. This is typically a positioning problem, when people stand normally their legs are a little spread apart and when liposuction is

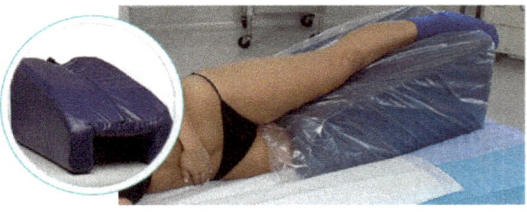

performed on the side of the hip, a bulge is present due to the positioning of the patient that does not properly reflect the natural contours of the body when standing. A special pillow is recommended when doing liposuction on the outer thigh (www.hksurgical.com)

The back portion of the thigh is another area that is commonly over corrected. This is an area that looks one way while laying down during the procedure, but when the patient is standing and leaning forward many times a dent can be evident.

The next few complications refer to problems in the skin:
8. Skin irregularity

Surface irregularities are covered in the section on loose skin but for completeness I will list it here as well. After lipo surface irregularities can be concerning to patients which can be caused by:

- overly aggressive lipo
- too superficial liposuction or the holes of the cannula were facing up to the under surface of the skin rather than down towards the deeper layers
- fibrosis with adhesions from failing to massage the areas after lipo
- inappropriate garment (most likely too tight)
- redundant skin/loose skin

This can be the result of improper liposuction but can also be the result of loose skin giving the appearance of irregular, non smooth skin. Again, fat is the glue between the skin and muscle. Imagine wearing a t shirt that is way too big for you. Instead of being able to tuck in the extra material into your pants (a tummy tuck), you need to have the extra material find a place on your body to rest passively. You are going to have areas where there is bunched up shirt. That is what happens with loose skin. If a tummy tuck is not going to be performed to remove the skin, it can get bunchy when it sticks back to the muscle and appear irregular.

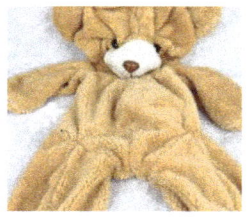

9. Skin laxity
Liposuction is a procedure that removes fat. It does not cause the skin to tighten. Skin tightening occurs as a result of the skin elasticity (90%) of the patient and post operative care at home (10%). There is no one, myself included, who can always predict how well your skin will retract back.

If you possess any of these criteria you are at risk of developing loose skin after liposuction, they include:
- stretch marks on the skin
- women who gave birth to a child
- women who gave birth to multiple children
- people who lost a significant amount of weight
- someone who is overweight with skin that can be pinched more than 1 inch
- genetic predisposition
- people who had massive weight loss surgery
- people over the age of 35
- Casusians are most at risk, followed by Asian and Latino

10. Asymmetry: Asymmetry can certainly happen, however I have seen many asymmetries that are present before surgery but are not noticed before surgery. No one is totally symmetric. Commonly, scoliosis can make one hip or should look higher than the opposite side creating a shifting of curves. It can make one side have a more snatched waistline than the other.

It is best for the doctor to point these things out before surgery. Sometimes they are not as noticeable when the patient is heavier, so they are missed before surgery.

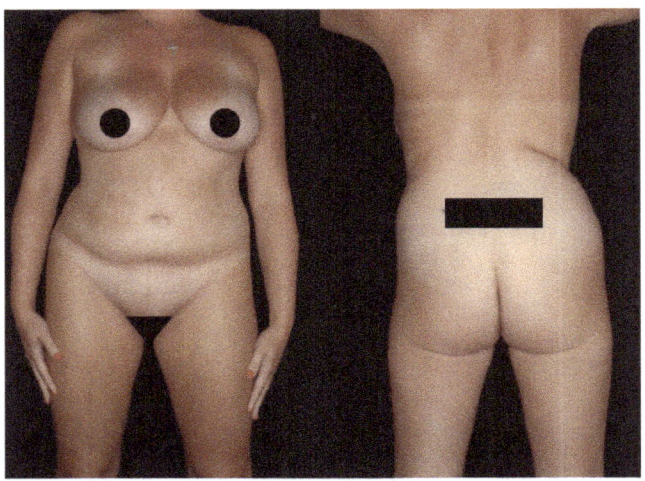

Patient with severe scoliosis. Creates asymmetries in the posture, waistline, butt shape, shoulder height and presented arm length. Many people have a much more subtle presentation. These differences are best discussed **before** surgery

11. Loose skin after liposuction can occur an any spot. Please check out in the chapter about skin if you are at risk and what can be done to minimize the chance of loose skin.

12. Liposuction holes that do not heal well. It is possible to get a slight depression from constant friction through the hole where liposuction took place, and even get a friction burn from the back and forth action of the cannula against skin. For that reason it is best to make the holes in hidden discrete areas. While doing liposuction I always put sterile lubrication ointment on the opening of the holes. The scarring of the access holes can potentially heal poorly as well, pigmented, thickened, hypertrophic or even keloid. many and where your doctor intends on placing your lipo holes. Find out how many and where your doctor intends on placing your lipo make sure they are in areas what can be hidden under your bra and underwear, and in the belly button. .

13. Skin hyperpigmentation

- Skin hyperpigmentation changes can occur following liposuction may be due to several factors such as:
- Hemosiderin deposition from ecchymosis
- Excessive pressure from compression garments
- Friction and shear at the incision site
- Sun exposure

- Exogenous drugs e.g., intramuscular iron therapy, contraceptive pills, minocycline etc

14. Skin necrosis is when the skin will actually become dark and die. This can be a small spot or a larger area where the blood supply to the corresponding skin has been compromised. This is most commonly occurring in smokers, over aggressive lipo, large seromas or hematomas, or lipo at the same time as a tummy tuck.

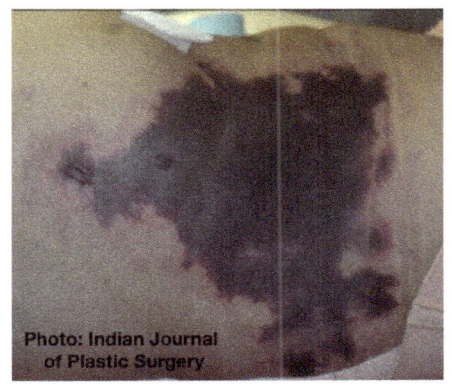
Photo: Indian Journal of Plastic Surgery

15. The butt bulge: This is an area of the skin of the butt that has herniated out in the form of a bulge. It is very rarely discussed in the literature and mentioned very minimally a few years ago refer to as a "blowout" of the butt. It can happen in a very constricted spot when the surgeon attempts to stretch this tight spot. This can also happen with aggressive massaging of the butt. Below is a picture of someone with a very tight spot on the lower corners of the butt that was attempted to stretch out. Which resulted in a herniation seen on the picture on the right. This is usually noted on the table during surgery. Oftentimes this is an area that becomes filled with serous fluid later and becomes a seroma or can be empty. This

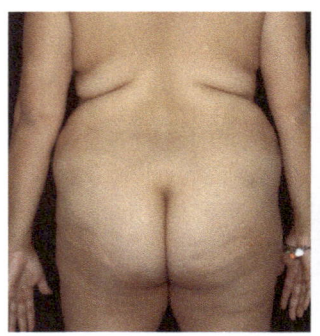
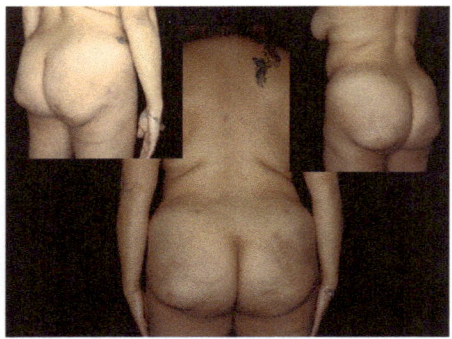

situation is verycomplicated to treat. It behaves similar to a broken spring on a mattress or a bubble on a tire. There is a soft bulge in the butt that almost appears empty.

Over time it fills with serous fluid (seroma) and requires multiple drainages. Over time the skin can actually stretch requiring a skin removal of the butt as well.

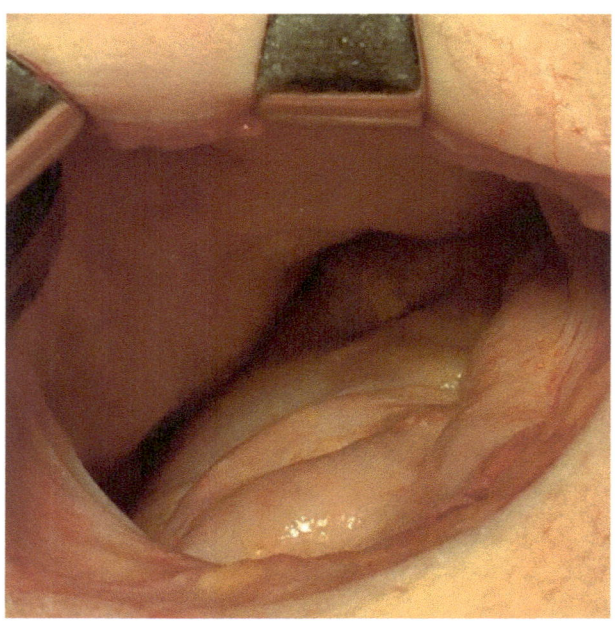

The above picture is a look inside the cavity of the seroma. As you can note, the walls are smooth and have a white fibrous coating. There is non blood supply to the inside of this space. any fat that enters into this space will not survive. This cavity must be obliterated or removed. Once the fluid is drained, one may attempt to address the cosmetic deformity that persists by injecting more fat. If the fat accidentally falls inside this space, the entire problem will reoccur.

The photo here shows what normal fresh fat looks like when it is harvested before a fat transfer. It is smooth and has a cream cheese consistency to it.

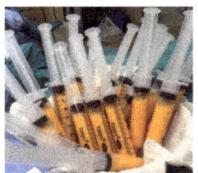

This is fat that was removed from the inside of the serum cavity. Clearly is is abnormal looking. The fat becomes hard and almost petrified. This is not viable fat that can survive but interestingly it doesn't break

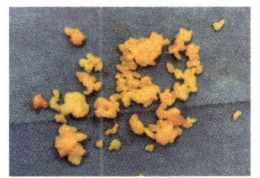

down into a creamy substance like much dead fat. Probably because the cells that would help break this fat down cannot access this cavity because there is no blood supply It turns into something that feels like popcorn kernels.

If an incision is needed to remove the redundant skin that has formed, it can usually be made in an inconspicuous areas that is not obnoxiously visible.

Those at risk include:

1. Caucasians
2. Thin skinned patients
3. Very flat areas most notable along the outside portion (lateral) of the butt

During a consultation many times I can anticipate these problems before they happen and I try to make this clear that there may be some areas that will not pop out. It is not as though I do not know how to pop them out, more like no one can pop these spots out. Areas that are tight sometimes so not respond nicely to expansion by fat addition.

I will show my patient he tight spot and demonstrate that the area when pinched does not pull away from the underlying tissue. This is shown in this picture. I will take a photo and show a patient so they can see what I see. When we pinch the skin the skin should take the shape of a "C", following the curve of the arch created by my first finger and thumb. If does not, it may not fully expand.

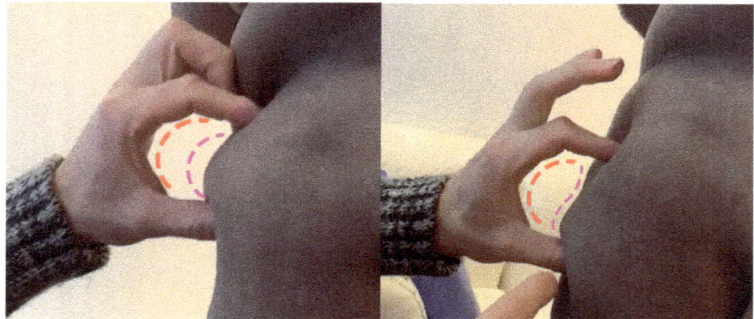

Sometimes it does surprise us, but there is a chance it will not and this spot will not be as expanded as we desire. If it is forced they will develop this complication and they will be more unhappy than they would with a booty that isn't fully 'poppin'.

This is a new complication that we are seeing as people are now wanting larger butts than ever before. There is no medical publications directly addressing this (it has been mentioned) however I have treated a few created by me and others from other doctors that did not know what to do. Our algorithm is effective and although it can take multiple interventions and a few months to treat it, it can eventually be treated to almost full correction.

To explain this phenomenon further, picture a yourself holding a piece of meatloaf from the top that represents the butt. Passing the injection cannula inside the meatloaf allows for fat deposits to be placed inside the butt. With each pass of the injection cannula the connections of the top layer to the bottom layer weakens. This allows for the

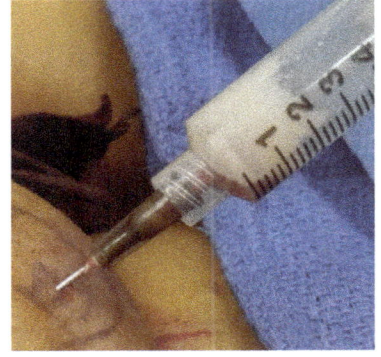

meatloaf to expand, for our example. In real life this allows the butt to expand. At some point a critical point can be reach where too many times the strokes back and forth have occurred and the meatloaf will become separated. That is what happens when the skin springs out. The question for the doctor is when is too many times? This is based on experience, weighing in the aforementioned risk factors, and having the maturity and experience to know when to stop.

Here is a diagram that explains the process.

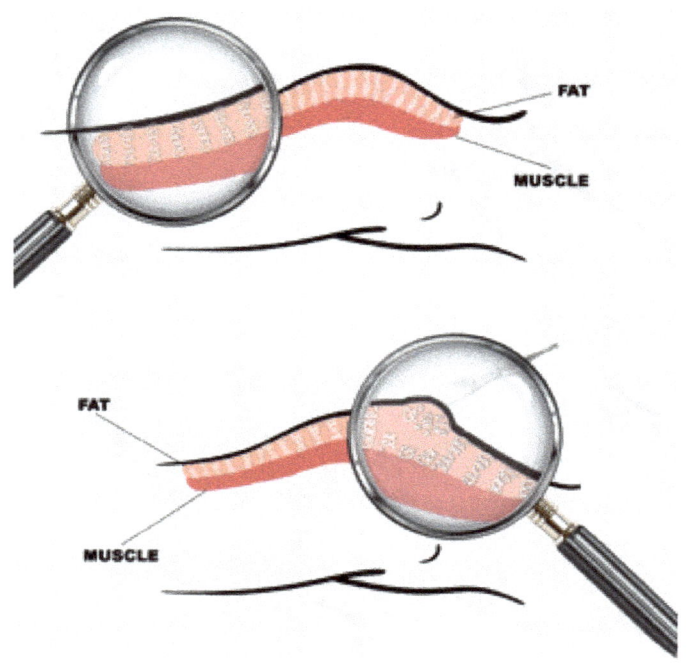

16. Pulmonary embolism is a scary complication and something you need to know about. Please read about it in the Chapters about the safety of the BBL.

17. Nodules and lumps/cysts
This can happen as a result of liposuction. They can be isolated areas of fat, or more commonly swelling or fibrosis after surgery. It is best to have lymphatic massage soon

after surgery to avoid this and to treat these areas as well. With aggressive massage these areas almost always resolve.

18. Nodules in the butt can occur in areas of fat transfer. These can be painful. This can happen when a large amount of fat is injected into the butt and a portion of the fat dies in a concentrated area that is too difficult for your own body to eliminate. To protect itself the body 'walls it off' and it creates a cyst.

In order for the fat to survive, blood vessels must come to the area to feed the fat with what it needs. When too much is in a spot, the blood vessels cannot penetrate the entirety of the fat collection. I often explain this to my patients with a frozen meatball. If you take a frozen meatball and put it in the microwave and heat it up. The outside will get hot but the inside may still be cold. This cold area is like the glob of fat that failed to get its blood supply. The fat cells die and liquify.

It can usually be treated pretty easily by having the patient point out the lump. With an 18 gauge needle, the cyst is aspirated leaving the wall of the cyst there but emptying out the dead liquified fat. It looks kid of like melted butter (not nice movie theatre yellow butter, more like the stick you use to make eggs) (I am quite hungry as I write this section, if you cant tell)

It is rare that an incision is needed to remove the cyst wall out but a very large one may require that.

If a large hard clump that has not liquefied has occurred the options for treatment include:
1. Do nothing- this is not dangerous but can be uncomfortable and annoying
2. continuing massaging it hoping to break it up and make it softer
3. Inject medications in it to allow it to get softer and potentially liquify (I use Kenalog and 5 Fluorouracil together
4. Make an incision to cut it out
5. Ultrasonic sound waves. In my office, Justo Concepcion PA, and I have been using this over the past 4 years or so and have had very nice success with it. Similar to how sound waves are used to break up kidney stones, we have been applying sound waves to the skin and softening/resolving these large hard plaques of dead fat. We are working on a publication as we speak.

19. My butt is too big. Is this even possible? This is rare, but has happened upon occasion. Making your vision clear with photos before surgery is a good idea. The words big, small, natural, are very subjective and your vision of these words may not match that of your surgeon. When it is too big, it can be liposuctioned carefully and conservatively as the skin of the butt often does not retract back well and it can leave the patient with loose, hanging skin in the butt.

Doing liposuction of the butt sounds intuitively simple. However, it is technique sensitive. The cannulas we used are straight and the butt is round. When the surgery is done the patient is laying down which distorts the presentation of the butt. When it is removed it is important to remove the fat without distorting the shape. I have done it with nice results but there is an art to it. It is a unique area to do liposuction, but being mindful of the shape while doing it can make for a nice result.

20. My butt is too small. Similarly, photos are helpful in creating your vision to match the doctors. This is more common than the other side of the spectrum. The limitations of the size one can reach is discussed in prior chapters.

21. The deep cuff A newer complication that we are now seeing is a deep crease under the butt of some women. This is happening from patients that desire a large butt, however their skin does not have the strength to support the weight of the newly enlarged butt and it starts to hang. It starts out looking excellent, then over a period of months and even years, the butt will fall. Much like a woman who has large breast implants, the skin will stretch as gravity takes its toll.

This patient often looks great naked or in a thong but complains that in some types of pants the butt shows a deepened crease that looks unnatural especially in the 3/4 rear view or performing an awkward leg up position, that I cannot imagine being too popular aside from some shaving poses.

How do I know if this is going to happen to me:
- People with loose skin are more predisposed to this
- Caucasian women
- stretched marked skin
- older patients (over age 50)
- those who lost a large amount of weight at one time
- smokers
- Ehlos Dandros disease or variant of the disease
- those with hyperextendable joints

I have corrected this before on patients using a variety of techniques alone or in combination with each other from skin excision, to lipo, J plasma® (Renuvion®), or Kybella® injections into the butt. Some are corrected to total perfection, while others see an improvement but still notice it a little bit.

Chapter 25: What to expect day 1 and early on

"Never did this before, that's what the virgin says
We've been generally warned, that's what the surgeon says"

Kanye West

The toughest thing about this surgery is the recovery period, no cap. It really tests what a patient can handle, and how dedicated your team is to helping you through this.

For you the patient, you need to handle:
- discomfort (sounds nicer than pain)
- this total body ache that people compare to getting hit by a car (thank god, i can't relate)
- disgusting feeling (leaking and wearing the same dirty garment)
- can't sit down, so now even more uncomfortable
- get sore from sleeping in the same position
- dizzy every time you get up or remove the garment
- with the pain meds you can get nauseous and constipated
- the embarrassment of looking like a slob in front of your caretaker

Sign me up! This isn't intended on talking you out of this, just to prepare you. You are going to need help, so do as much as you can BEFORE the surgery to prepare and choose your care taking team wisely.

The caretaker needs to handle:

- to be at your beckon call for food and getting up
- getting the garment on and off
- dealing with the inevitable stink of healing
- helping hold the urinal while peeing, often we have heard of friends helping clean one's ass. I think I would personally find a way to do this myself, but people have gotten help
- dispense any medications
- deal with the moaning
- be there to physically support the patient while ambulating
- drive the patient around for at least 10 days
- not panic

You deserve a metal for this. Especially if you are cleaning your friend's ass.

The first night

For many patients this will be a blur. You haven't eaten all day, and the only thing you have taken in is iv fluid. This fluid however isn't in your belly, it was put in your veins, however it is now leaking into your injured body to contribute to swelling. You need to drink a lot over the next few days. Whatever you normally drink you probably need double.

You are going to be leaking fluid. This fluid will look like blood. Imagine a bathtub filled with water and then adding a few drops of dyes. The bathwater changes color. Your doctor is likely using tumescent fluid injected under the skin. It mixes with a little bit of blood and looks like a lot of blood is

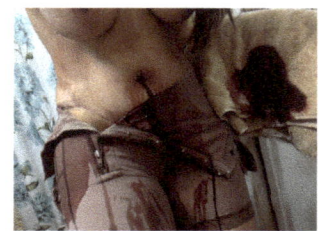

pouring out of your liposuction holes. Here is a typical picture of what the fluid looks like staining the garment. You should contact your doctor if you are concerned. Your doctor who took care of you should know what is normal for you moreso than the emergency room, your friend, or google.

Tonight I want my patients to lay in bed and do not try to get up for anything, aside for a fire or a sale at the Gucci store.

Your goals tonight should be:
1. Pee just off the bed
2. drink

When you have to pee it should be done as demonstrated similar to the photo shown here. You can actually leave your faja on and use the access hole in the 'pee pee' spot to sneak the urinal in. As you can see this is usually a two person job, as the gentleman in the photo appears to be quite helpful.

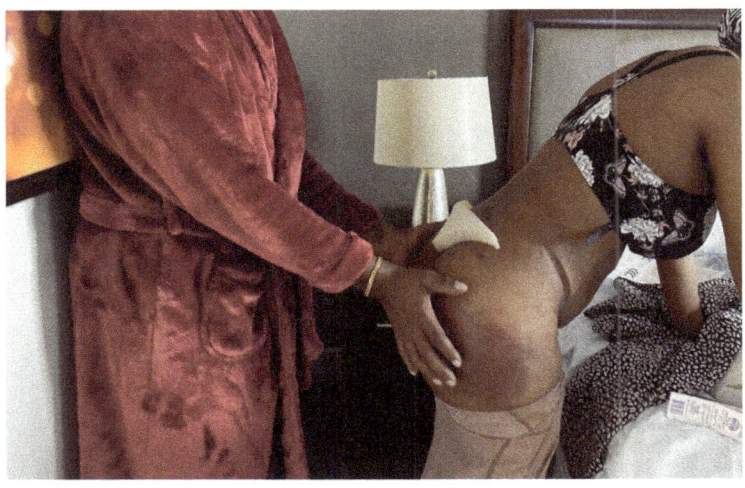

Try to open the flaps in the crotch area in the garment wide enough for the urinal to fit in. Often patients pee on themselves and this can get kind of nasty with no garment to change into. Additionally, laying in a garment with pee in the groin will cause a burn-like rash in between the legs, that can be quite irritating. Similar to a diaper rash.

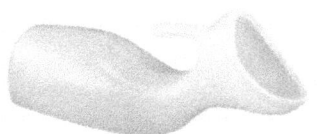

We do not recommend walking to the bathroom on the evening after surgery. We have had patients get dizzy while walking and fainting, injuring themselves in the process. After the first night most people can walk to the bathroom and pee using the suggestions shown in the Chapter 26, dedicated to going to the bathroom.

You should drink very bland things at first: chicken broth, tea, water, gatorade. If you can tolerate eating food, the foods should again be very plain: toast, rice, chicken, yogurt, or cottage cheese.

Whatever recommendations your doctor had with regard to medications follow them. My patients generally take an antibiotic pill before bed and a pain medication pill.

POST OPERATIVE DAYS 2 AND 3

The drainage is still coming out but significantly less. The arms may still be draining a bit more. The dizziness you had last night is better and you will still feel it when you get up too fast, or when you take off the garment. These days are the worst. Stay strong. After the third day, things start to improve.

Goals today include:
1. sponge bath
2. change dirty absorptive pads
3. drink A LOT!
4. eat protein rich meals
5. Walk around a little with assistance
6. we advise our patients to keep the stockings on today

After day three I allow my patients to remove the garment to take a shower. Someone needs to be with you and this needs to happen very slowly. Other chapters go more into detail about fainting. But please be aware, when the garment comes off, your blood pressure will drop and you will feel dizzy and could faint. Fainting is not a crisis in that of itself, but falling and hurting yourself can be. Take the garment off super slowly. Unhook a few hooks and wait a minute or two, then continue. Taking off the garment should take 10 minutes or so to do it safely.

Keep in mind this is the turning point of the recovery process. Tomorrow you will start to slowly feel better.

POSTOPERATIVE DAY 7 (1 WEEK)

This is the day I usually see our patients in the office. Most of these patients are still quite pale and weak. Their lips are dusky in color and the whites of their eyes can be a little yellow.

The pain is tolerable however they are still quite sore and stiff. If you haven't gotten a lymphatic massage yet, this is a great day to do so. You should have pooped already. If you have not take an enema. More about dropping a poo in the next chapter.

Today in the office if there are any remaining dissolve sutures (stitches) I remove them. Their job is essentially done and by removing them the scars will heal better and people complain about the sutures getting caught on the material of the garment. People get nervous that the suture removal is painful. It is not. It's simply cutting the string, like cutting a piece of hair.

Don't be concerned if your butt is hard. It will get softer over the next week or two. Cellulite that you may have had before the surgery may appear to be gone. This is due to swelling, expect it to come back as the swelling subsides. Today you should also be examined for potential seromas. This is something your doctor will do and drain if necessary. Seromas are covered in multiple chapters.

POSTOPERATIVE DAY 10

This is a milestone day because this is the day the fat in your butt has started to stabilize and find its home. This is the day we ask our patients to remove their foam on their lower back above their butt. For my oatients, the foam is sticking to the back with a very good glue. Please DO NOT rip the foam off. Let it get wet and take it off slowly, or use coconut oil to get it off. You can take it off in shower but cutting the foamy part and working the glue off. We have had patients rip it off and it can leave a discoloration of the skin that can be long lasting and even permanent. Today is the day we allow our patients to sit on their boppy/booty pillows. Your doctor may have their own advice.

POSTOPERATIVE DAY 14

This is the day most of our patients return to work. If you have a desk job this should not be an issue. If you have a job that entails manual work, you may need to prolong your revery period or return with light duties.

All movements should be made like a robot. If you need something high above your head, it is best to get someone else to get it. Otherwise, use a step stool to not allow your arm to stretch your body. Although the tightness may make you want to stretch to counter it, but it is a bad idea. The fat was removed from your body and that was the glue attaching your skin to the muscles. the early attachment process occurs on the 10th day and your stretching can overpower the attachment. If this happens you can get a fluid collection in the space (seroma) or the skin can be loose. Similarly, if you need something from the ground bend at your knees and don't stretch down to get it.

For example, we had a patient driving her car 2 weeks out and she needed something from their back seat. She reached behind her while driving and felt what she described as a light pop. The next day she called with a fluid collection that required us to drain her on 3 separate occasions in the office. It is an easy procedure that requires nothing more than local anesthesia and a few minutes but is better if avoided. It is more of a nuisance than a complication.

MONTHS AFTER SURGERY

We do have patients that complain of some tenderness when running when their butt bounces around. Eventually this does go away but can take beyond a year.

We do have very few patients who notice that there are a couple spots of an altered sensation of the skin. From liposuction alone we have not seen total numbness but some people do have a spot here or there where the sensation can be less than normal or even altered. For example, itching the bottom part of your belly, you may feel the itch instead on the upper portion of your body. If these things do occur, they are very minor concerns to the patient and never have I heard of it as a major problem.

Although the majority of swelling has subsided after 3 month (90-95%), your last bit of swelling can linger for quite a while. Especially those who have had other prior abdominal surgeries including prior lipo. Time is the best remedy. Lymphatic massage can still help. Even though you are not required to wear a faja anymore, it will not hurt to continue. If you are having one of those days where you feel you are swollen put the faja on. Avoid salt. Exercise can actually help make the swelling go away quicker. Some patents have reported success from Calendula tea three times daily. Some also report dandelion root, which comes in a pill form from the health food store, can be helpful as a mild diuretic also.

Chapter 26: Going to the bathroom

> "For about a month my urine smelled like marshmallows."
> *Will Ferrell*

It sounds silly but it can be a major issue. Constipation is unfortunately fairly common and a huge pain in the ass- literally. The pain from constipation is often worse than pain from the actual surgery. This is from a host of factors:
1. Narcotics - the pain medications used will slow motility of the gut
2. The garment after surgery slows gastrointestinal motility.
3. Lack of mobility will slow bowel function
4. Dehydration -
    a. before surgery you haven't eaten since midnight the night before
    b. During surgery you lose blood and volume
    c. After surgery your appetite is less
    d. Nausea may deter you from eating or drinking

Imagine being constipated, trying to maneuver yourself to the bathroom in pain, trying to poop either through the hole in the garment or getting the garment off, not sitting on the bowl, having your loved one right outside the door or in the room with you, nice picture we just painted, no?

It is so important to drink a lot! Set small goals for yourself, like one bottle of Poland Spring every hour. In addition to the need for hydration because of fat lost, the body produces a hormone known as cortisol. This is a stress hormone who's production goes up as a result of surgery. The amount produced during surgery is equal to that if you stood in the middle of a highway, and allowed a truck to come full speed and stop right before hitting you. The way your body perceives surgery is a major assault on your body, that you do not flee from. These cortisol levels not only slow digestion but increase your fluid requirements even more than your regular baseline requirements.

We recommend taking stool softeners a few days BEFORE surgery to keep everything regular throughout your healing process. The liquid version of milk of magnesia is our laxative of choice. Some people like Colace or even drink prune juice, whatever works for you it fine.

If you are regularly constipated it is best to try to correct this before surgery. Take fiber supplements, and a mild laxative (Senakot®) before surgery. If you cannot go 3 days or so after surgery I would try to back off of the narcotics and use over the counter meds. Pooping should be a priority about now and you should consider an enema.

There are many different approaches to conquer constipation, to summarize them you can:

take a fiber supplement	calcium polycarvophil (fiberCon), methyl cellulose (Citrucel), Psyliium (Metamucil, Konsyl)

eat fiber	rice, beans, fruits and vegetables, while grain breads or cereals, and oats
drink water	
take a laxative stimulant	senna-sennosides (senokot), bisacodyl (Dulcolax, Ducodyl, Correctol)
take an osmotic laxative	lactulose (Kristalose), polyethylene glycol (MiraLAX), magnesium citrate, magnesium hydroxide (Phillips Milk of Magnesia)
as your doc for a script	polyethylene glycol (Golytely, Nulytely)
lubricant laxative	mineral oil
stool softener	docusate sodium (Colace) or docusate calcium (Surfak),
take an enema	sodium phosphate (Fleet), soapsuds, and tap water enemas
use a suppository	glycerin or bisacodyl suppository
walk around	increases the blood supply to your intestines
massage the belly	deep massage of the belly will stimulate the bowels, many people after they get they lymphatic massage will unload.

When it's time to go #2:

1. Different patients have shared different techniques. The goal is to not sit down on the bowl to potentially distort

the butt. I would recommend taking the garment off rather than trying to poop through the hole in the garment. Some people have placed a stack of towels on the front edge of the bowel to avoid sitting down.

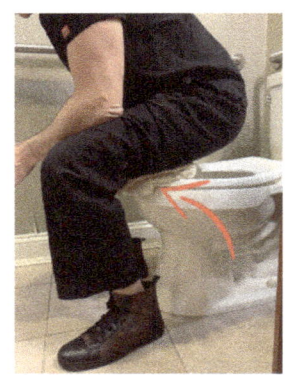

2. Others have had success with a simple squat.

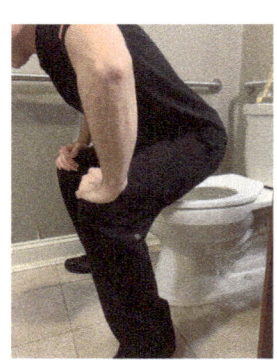

3. Others place a chair in front of the toilet. Patients have used a folding snack table for support as well.

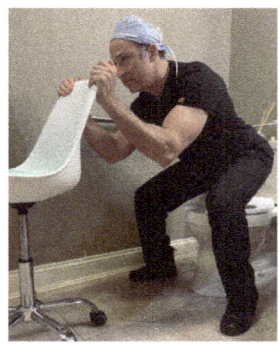

4. Some find success squatting reversed on the toilet and holding on to the toilet bowl tank for stability.

5. Some patients have just put a wee wee pad down and peed, like a puppy. Ya. I said that, and I am not demonstrating that.

While there is a hole in the garment for going to the bathroom, unless you are a former fighter pilot with amazing aim, you are best taking the garment off; even to pee. The first night is an exception to the rule.

I would not try to take the garment off the first night. I would use a handheld urinal. This can be purchased on Amazon, of course. If you do not have one you can use a plastic bag while

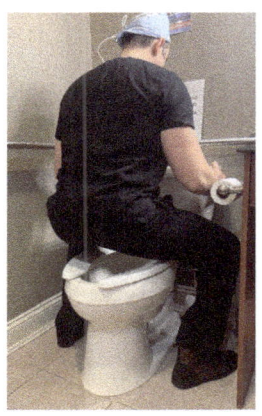

leaning over the side of the bed. The reason we recommend using the hole on the first day is because it is difficult to get up and ambulate the first night. Many patients do complain of dizziness and some do faint. The next day, people start to feel better with their strength.

We have had people fearful of taking the garment off and believe they have good enough aim to pee through the hole in the garment. A little mist of urine can continuously get on the garment. Urine is an acid (uric acid) and can cause a burn like reaction on the skin. This is very common with babies getting diaper rash.

It is often embarrassing for a patient when they realize that this was the cause and is handled delicately. The rash resolves with the garment being removed and washed and usually we use a cream like Silvadene over the skin. Full resolution of the skin takes place in a week or two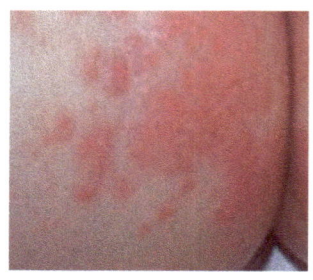
(picture of typical rash from urine burn-dermatitis)

After the first night it is again my recommendation to remove the garment to pee. If you are having trouble squatting or sitting as described you can take the garment off and enter the shower. You can pee in the shower to avoid the entire siting process.

Chapter 27: Sitting

"Be humble, sit down"
Kendrick Lamar

You will never realize what a luxury sitting is until after this surgery. Let me first say, there is no direct scientific evidence that says, you should not sit for "x" amount of time. This is based on my personal experience of doing thousands of Brazilian Butt Lifts and seeing that many people through the healing process. Some people sat too early, others waited varying amounts of times, and some probably still haven't sat because they are afraid to mess things up. By also applying basic rules of healing that has been studied from other types of surgery, we can extrapolate a timetable for sitting after this procedure.

Very rarely is any pressure good for your butt. The only exception to the rule is if someone's fat has shifted early after surgery and the fat is sitting too high. This sometimes happens when someone lays or sits in the wrong position, most commonly on patients who

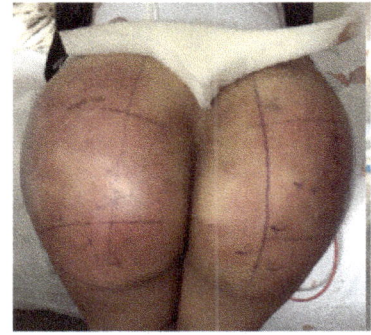

have had a tummy tuck and a BBL. Many of these patients will look very "top heavy" on the butt, however in a few weeks this can be manipulated down.

Although there has never been a peer reviewed medical publication showing sitting to be detrimental to your BBL result, trust me, it is. My recommendation is not to sit at all for the first 10 days. The reason I chose 10 days as my number is because it has been seen in brow lift surgery that it takes 10 days to form early scar tissue and skin adhesion. It is my belief this scar tissue creates almost a net to keep the fat from shifting. During this time I place a foam triangle above the top of the butt crack. This serves 3 functions:
1. It reminds you not to sit down
2. If you do sit it prevents the fat from shifting into the lower back. (fat resides in the subcutaneous plane under the skin. This plane is connected to the areas where lipo was performed. If pressure is applied to the butt the fat will follow the path of least resistance and travel in the empty areas where fat was removed) this foam acts as a mechanical barrier. (for more information on this check out Chapter 33)
3. It allow the skin on the lower back to 'stick' to the bone. This area we want totally devoid of fat. That 'lordotic' back look is very nice and often requested during the surgery. The foam helps create that.

After day 10 it is ok to sit.

Rules of sitting:
1. This sitting should be on a 'boopy pillow' or one of the other commercial booty pillows available. It could be "the booty buddy", the "Dr Miami booty pillow", or whatever else you want to use. The purpose of this pillow should be to have it 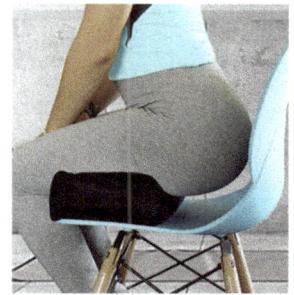 positioned under the hamstrings and to keep the butt almost in the air. It should not contact the seat cushion. Very light touching is ok. Some patients love this, others complain that it is too hard on their hamstrings. Some patients use this to drive and a soft pillow to sit.

If the foam is too boujee for you, you can go to Bed Bath and Beyond and grab a boppy pillow. Leave the opening to the back and sit on this. Make sure you use your 20% off coupon post card. If you don' have one, check your neighbor's mailbox. I have never seen someone pay full price at that store. Don't try the neck pillow from the airport.

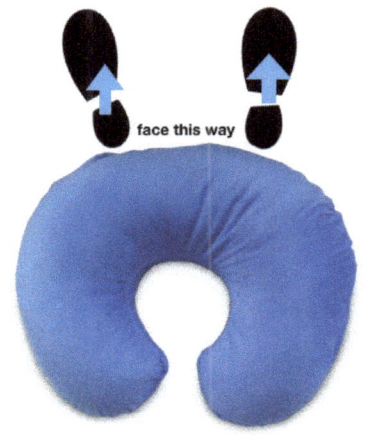

If your ass fits in that, ask your doctor for a refund.

2. When you put pressure on skin, the skin turns white. This is because the blood supply is temporarily routed away from this area. We want as much blood supply to the butt as possible to allow for the fat to thrive. Just like a skin graft, a kidney transplant, or any transfer of tissue we need a healthy blood supply to the recipient site. When sitting I would try to not sit for more than 30 minutes at a time. Stand up for a few minutes and let the blood flow back to the butt. If you are driving, pull over and stand up for a bit. Reposition the pillow a bit so you are not in the same position all day. Lean on one side more than another for a while then rotate to the other side.

3. This is especially true for those who are bus/taxi drivers, or those with a desk job. Even after healing is complete try to minimize the same position all day, every day to maintain your results and protect that investment.

If you don't believe me, look at those in a nursing home. True, many of the elderly are nutritionally and health compromised but bed sores are a common problem. Bedsores are from someone's own body weight (laying, not even standing!) putting pressure on a spot on a soft mattress! Being in the same position for a prolonged period of time will eventually cause the skin to break down. Then the fat and muscle can eventually be eroded exposing bone! I am not suggesting you will erode a hole in your body by sitting after surgery but pressure, in the same position over a prolonged amount of time is definitely detrimental to your results.

We ask you use this pillow for at least 8 weeks. After 8 weeks we usually give the ok sleep on your back as well.

I will say, we have seen some of our long term follow ups who stop by the office or post some IG pictures up who look beyond amazing. I have asked these women, even a year after surgery, "when did you start sitting on your butt". Their response has often been, "Still waiting".

Chapter 28: Sleeping

"I think sleeping was my problem in school. If school had started at 4 pm , I'd be a college graduate today."
George Foreman

This is probably one of the most difficult parts of the recovery process. We do not want any pressure on your butt. The more you stay off it, the better. Unwanted pressure can shift the fat early on in the process, and can decrease the blood supply to the fat and cause more fat to die.

You are going to make a mess on your bed. You could potentially ruin your mattress as well. This is not the time to wear your sexy pajamas and your 5000 count Egyptian cotton sheets. Get some shitty sheets from Walmart and get a plastic mattress cover. You will have fluid leaking out of you, through your clothes, and everywhere for probably 3 days or so. Don't dress like Kim K going to the Hamptons, don't wear white!

<u>LIPO 360 /BBL</u>
You should be sleeping on your belly. For those not used to this, it may be hard to stay asleep or fall asleep. Be sure to explain this specifically to your doctor and they can prescribe the appropriate medication. There are medications that can be given to help you fall asleep, and others that can make you stay asleep. Not like MJ, safely. Some people complain of lower back discomfort. Sometimes a pillow under your shins can alleviate some of the discomfort.

Lipo 360/BBL with a surgery on the front (breast, tummy tuck, etc)

For the person who had surgery on their butt and their front (like breasts or a tummy tuck), they cannot sleep on their belly or their back. With liposuction of the stomach is ok to sleep on your belly.

These are the options:

1. My first choice for these people is always sleeping on their side. You may have had fat transferred to your hips so you should not put weight directly on your side. Every time you wake up during the night switch to the other side.

When we stand up all the weight is on our feet.

However when we are on our side, 100% of your weight is not on your hip. It is distributed across your entire side of the body touching the soft bed.
So, if you do happen to put some pressure on the hip, we have not seen this negatively affect your result.

You can get a full body pregnancy pillow and sleep on the front part of your hip which should have no impact on your result. Typically fat is added to the side of the hip to create a nice curve but the front part of the hip is not as critical.

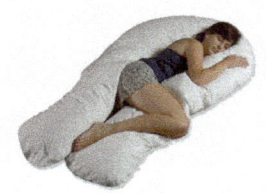

Most of my patients start off their recovery after surgery all ready to go, wanting to do everything "by the book". After a few days, their feelings change when their hips are starting to hurt and they no longer can tolerate this position.

2. If you are miserable sleeping on your side, you can sleep inside an inner tube.

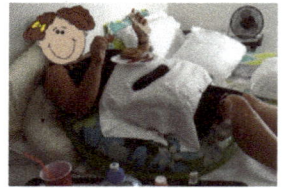

Yes, the same tube you have seen in the lazy river or your swimming pool. Just make sure it is big enough to fit your butt in it. You will need to put some pillows behind your back to support you.

For some, their butt won't fit in the tube hole or they still can't get comfortable. If you have firm pillows (maybe from your sofa) you can create a fortress of pillows to bring that butt in the air. this may be harder to do if you

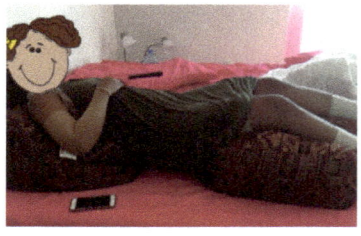

had a tummy tuck too. your tummy tuck will require you

so keep your stomach flexed at 30 degrees and I personally do not think it is great for your butt to have that bend in your back, stretching and putting that much pressure on the skin on the butt and legs and potentially shifting the fat (like a pimple ready to blow) and creating so much pressure that restricts blow flow.

3. You can cut a hole in a beach chair.

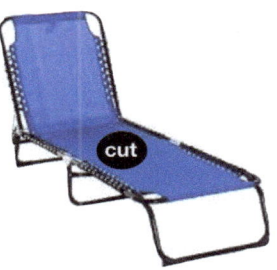

4. There are air mattresses that are made for this surgery with a hole in the middle. We have heard negative feedback from a few of our patients who have tried it. Some have complained they had a hard time getting out of the hole once getting positioned in it. They are very similar to pregnancy mattresses with holes in the mattress if you are having a hard time finding one. It is nice in that it is easy to clean, but the feedback from most of our patients who have tried this is not favorable.

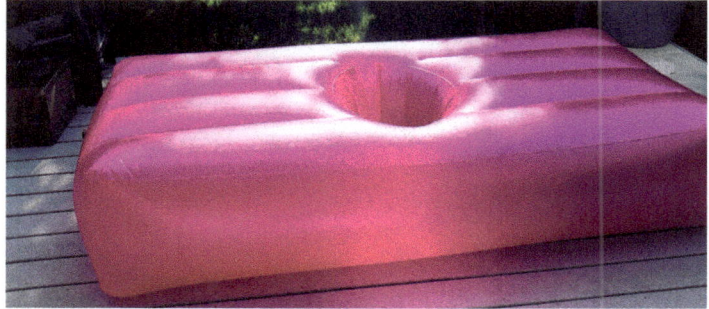

If you had a straight up BBL without any surgery on your front (aside from the lipo) your sleeping is pretty straight forward. Take the advice of 2 Live Crew, sleep "face down, ass up".

Sweet dreams :)

Chapter 29: Eating

"For me, skinny is just a style of jeans, not a goal."
Kim Kardashian

People commonly ask what to eat after surgery to get their optimal results.

Somewhere on the internet people are reading to eat fatty foods to 'feed the fat' in their butt. This idea is nonsense to me. If you want to target your diet to address what your body is craving after surgery it should focus on:

1. Protein: Your body requires protein to heal itself. It the basic building block of muscle and tissue. This can come in the form of fish, meat, chicken, tofu, or even protein shakes.
2. Iron: As a result of aggressive liposuction you will like have a transient anemia. It takes 120 days for a new red blood cell to form so it may take a while to get those numbers up again. You will likely look a little pale, especially in your lips and whites of your eyes. Your hands may feel cold and you may be weak and dizzy. Iron will help those numbers go up faster. A supplement is certainly an option. Taking an iron supplement can have side effects. I recommend a slow release iron like Slow Fe or Ferro sequel to avoid nausea and constipation.

There are two types of iron: heme iron and non heme iron. Heme iron is absorbed better to replenish hemoglobin.

Red meats, fish, and poultry all contain heme and non heme iron. Plant base iron sources are generally rich in non heme iron. It is more difficult for your body to increase iron levels while eating non heme iron.

Good sources of iron include: beef, lamb, ham, turkey, chicken, veal, pork, dried beef, liver, liverwurst, eggs (any style).

Non heme sources include: Iron-fortified breakfast cereals, rice, breads and pastas, cooked beans and lentils, tofu, pumpkins, squash or sesame seeds, chickpeas, kidney beans and lima beans, dried apricots, baked potatoes, nuts, broccoli stems, raw and cooked spinach and kale, and peas.

3. low salt foods It is best to avoid salty foods after surgery. It will create fluid retention which will prolong swelling after surgery and may increase your risk of getting a seroma.

4. LOTS OF WATER Your body needs a lot of water to replenish and heal itself. You just had a large amount of fat removed from your body, that creates fluid shifts that require water to balance out. You lost blood. Your fluid has leaked into your tissue to create swelling. You did not eat all day because of your surgery requirements. You need water!!!! It is not uncommon to get a severe headache a day or two after surgery because of dehydration. Also a low grade fever can be a result of dehydration.

The *night after surgery* you should eat whatever you feel like you can tolerate. This is not the night to turn over a new leaf and start eating what you are not accustomed to. Comfort foods that are bland are ideal. Things like tea, toast, crackers, chicken soup are all good and easy on the stomach after a full day without eating, allowing the drugs on board to slowly wear off.

It is many times difficult to eat days after surgery. The garment you are wearing it likely tight on your stomach. You cannot sit like a normal person at a table to eat. You are nauseous from the pain medications you are taking. You cannot cook for yourself. For all of these reasons many times you may not be eating as much as you normally do. I will say your calorie requirements are actually higher in the healing period than normally. For that reason, I do recommend eating to 'feed the fat'. However I am not a believer in eating bad foods to keep the fat cells happy.

    As a general rule, a proper and balanced diet will prevent a lot of the weight gain that occurs with unhealthy eating habits. In order to maintain good results after liposuction, you should incorporate more fruits, vegetables, whole grains, and lean protein into your diet, while reducing the intake of sugars, simple carbohydrates, and saturated fats. Eating several smaller meals throughout the day will help maintain your energy levels and keep you from feeling deprived between meals.

    Frequent hydration is also important. Drinking a sufficient amount of water during the day helps control hunger, maintains a healthy metabolism, and aids in digestion. Although liposuction can dramatically improve the contours of your body, it is not magic. You can still gain weight after liposuction if you return to your old, unhealthy eating habits.

That being said, there are some of my colleagues who believe eating certain foods can increase the chance for fat cell survival. Above I have listed the things I believe are important to get you healing quickly and getting you back into your normal routine. I am not fully sure if eating certain foods after surgery help maintain the BBL results but it cannot hurt.

Dr. Myoussef in a group message I am included in, shared the foods the he has seen a benefit from below:

eggs	avacado	salmon
fat cheese (yellow)	nuts, almonds, all types of oilseeds (Can be included in salad)	shrimp
milk cream	peanut butter	olive oil
if you want to eat bread or pizza that is made of almond or coconut flour cut cow's milk and include coconut or almond milk		

Chapter 30: Showering

*"Hot damn, hot water, hot shower
Hotlanta, smoking green, cauliflower."*
Chance the Rapper

I advise my patients to sponge bathe for the first three days. It is common to leak for the first few days from the liposuction holes. The gauze should be replaced as much as necessary. Many patients will want to take off the garment to wash. Please check out the next chapter on how to care for your garment.

Generally I give the ok to shower on the 3rd day. The reason why, being the first few days your blood pressure will likely not be stable enough to allow you to take off the garment and then take a hot shower. By day 3, you should be ok to do so (not to mention any time longer without a shower you would probably smell so bad you may vomit).

1. Take the garment off slowly. When going from laying to a standing position this too should be done slowly. If you want to wash your garment now, you can give it a quick rinse. I would not wait for it to dry before replacing it.
2. Take a shower with someone in the bathroom. If you have a friend or a sibling who you do not want to see you naked, sing while in the shower so when the singing stops, they should come in. Do not lock the bathroom door.

3. It is ok to get the wounds wet and any adherent foam wet. Just pat everything dry. Any antibacterial soap is a good idea. I do not like the Hibiclens for daily showers. It is quite tough on the skin and should only be used before surgery and under your doctors advice.
4. If you need to pee, now is a good time to do it.
5. Don't go too hot! Your skin could be a little numb and you may burn yourself accidentally. Additionally if the shower is too hot, you can potentially faint.

Chapter 31: Cleaning the faja

"It's sweet that I don't have to do my own laundry."
Adam Levine

For the rookies out there, a faja is a supportive post surgical garment.
The first few days after surgery your faja is going to get filthy. You will be leaking blood tinged fluid from the lipo holes. We generally recommend taking it off to wash duding your first shower on the third day.

Taking the garment before than can:

1. Cause you to faint. When the garment comes off, your blood pressure will come down and you could pass out. By the third recovery day the sensation may be better than earlier on.
2. Make it very difficult to get it back on. You will swell quite a bit for the first 72 hours after surgery. If you take it off to wash then dry the garment you will have time to swell and it can be very difficult to get it back on.

Exceptions to this rule are:
1. you pee on yourself. If trying to pee through the hole at the bottom of the faja you may get it on yourself. Not only does it feel gross to lay in your own urine, but a

very nasty rash can develop with the acidity of the urine versus the delicate thin skin of the inner thighs.
2. if you have a second garment. you can take it off to immediately put the new one on.

If you need to take it off and don't have a second one, give it a quick rinse. Wring it out and put it back on damp. Someone can use a hair drier on cold air while you are showering to dry it off a little. You should not wait for it to completely dry.

When it is time to wash your faja/garment take it off slowly. The removing process should take at least 5 minutes to slowly allow the blood pressure to equilibrate. If you feel dizzy sit. You don't want to pass out and hurt yourself. Have someone with you.

Once it is off, wash it in cold water and Oxyclean. If you don't like Oxyclean you can use 1 tablespoon of peroxide with a gallon of water.

Allow it to air dry. Putting it in the drier will shrink it too much and you have no shot at getting its back on.

You certainly don't want to smell horrible and lay in your own filth: the increased chance of infection, you will feel miserable, and no one will want to help you because of your stink. On the same token, don't be too concerned to be looking your finest. People understand, you just had surgery.

Chapter 32: I'm gonna faint!

"I brought my bitch to the bank, then she passed out."
Quavo

After this surgery, especially that first night, it is not uncommon to feel dizzy and some people can even faint (syncope). This should still be brought to the attention of your doctor. This is likely from a drop in blood pressure and a failure of your body to maintain blood flow to the brain.

When your heart beats, it pumps blood around your body to delivery the oxygen and energy it needs. As this blood moves it pushes against the sides of the blood vessels. The strength of this pushing force is your blood pressure. It is measured with a blood pressure cuff.

<u>Contributing factors to you feeling faint include:</u>

1. when the fat is removed your body tries to accommodate for this tissue loss by a process called 'fluid shifts' which can lower your blood pressure
2. bleeding during surgery
3. not eating or drinking before surgery causing you to already start your healing process 'behind' your normal requirements
4. some people get queasy or light headed by the sight of the blood tinged fluid
5. The garment helps sustain your blood pressure and when it comes off you can get light headed and faint. When it comes off you get decompression of the lower extremities which can drop your blood pressure.

6. The anesthesia and medications in your system can contribute to a lower blood pressure

Preventive measures for fainting include
1. when peeing for at least the first 24 hours, use a female urinal through the holes in your garment,
2. Stand up slow after urinating
3. when the garment comes off do it slowly with assistance. Undo a few hooks wait a moment of two then a few more, etc.
4. do not remove the garment on an empty stomach
5. have someone with you when showering for the first time
6. so not lock the bathroom when using the bathroom
7. Do not be scared of seeing blood stained clothing. The more leaking out, the less bruising and swelling in the long run.

The first signs of fainting include a feeling of lightheadedness or dizziness. Your skin may become pale, clammy, and damp. Perspiration may occur and pupils may dilate. Weakness and confusion is soon to follow.

If this feeling has started it is important to clear an area so if the person falls they do not injure themselves. Call for help. Have the patient lay down on their back and elevate their feet. This is not the time to worry about the butt getting 'ruined' a moment or so should not alter one's long term results and this medical problem should take precedent. A cool compress should be helpful on the neck or forehead. If you have ammonia or alcohol, placing some on a cotton ball and hold it under the patient's nose.

Fainting is a process that should correct itself and is self limiting. The biggest fear of actually fainting is inuring your head or neck when falling. If you are feeling faint or have fainted after surgery let your doctor know immediately. If you have a tendency to faint, tell your doctor before surgery.

Chapter 33: Garments

"Opinions are like assholes, everyone has one, and they usually stink."
Mr. Sessa, My High school Golf Coach 1991

The topic of garments (faja) is probably the most (believe it or not) "argued" about topic in our office. Patients have very very strong opinions about the type of garment they should be using. Their information usually comes online, or from some insta-famous person with a sick body that probably is lying about the work she had done, or is photoshopped/facetuned. Others have spoken to someone who is from a Latin American country and 'knows better'. It is a leap of faith for some people to trust their doctor, but if you trusted them to do the surgery, my advice is trust them to manage your care after. No one has more experience doing the surgery, no one has more knowledge of what went down in the operating room, what limitations or challenges they encountered during the surgery, and no one has had the opportunity to evaluate your skin from the inside aside from your doctor.

I have seen post operative garments absolutely ruin surgical outcomes. There are very few times I have seen post operative garments save a surgery. That being said, here are my guidelines to proper garment wearing.

Benefits of a properly fitting garment include:

Keeping swelling to a minimum
Allow for proper skin retraction
Minimize chance of seroma
Comfort
Can help shape the butt in some rare situations

Potential hazards of the wrong garment:
Irregularity of skin
Burns of skin
Indentations
Shrinking the butt
rashes
distorting the belly button

TOO TIGHT IS NOT GOOD!
A major misconception about post operative garments is, the tighter the better. There are people who believe that a tighter garment will better remove the swelling from the belly. THIS IS NOT TRUE. To understand why it is important to understand some basic anatomy.

In the body there are 3 major types of vessels (shown in the diagram are various cross sections. This is like taking a straw, cutting it in half then looking down the hole)

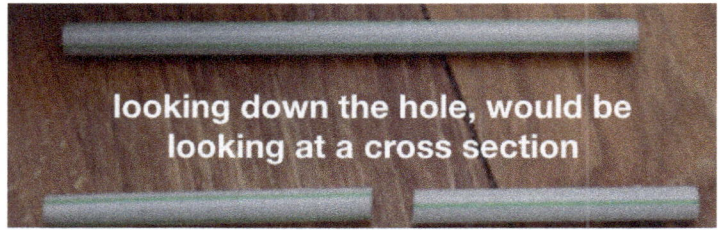

Arteries carry oxygenated blood away from the heart. Of the three aforementioned types of vessels its walls are the thickest. Blood flows through the arteries because of a pump pushing blood through them, This pump is the heart.

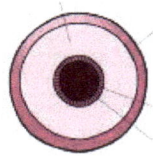

Veins carry deoxygenated blood to the heart. These vessel walls are less firm than an artery but still have some strength to them. That is where an IV (intravenous) line goes. There is not a direct pump in a vein but there are valves in the vein that prevent backflow.

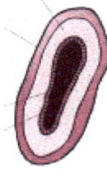

Arteries and veins are a closed system meaning the blood cells are constantly within a vessel. The lymphatic system is an open system. It recruits its fluid from the space between the cells when pressure pushes fluid between the cells to enter the system.

Lymphatic vessels carry lymphatic fluid. This is where swelling presents itself. These vessels are very flimsy and weak. There is very low pressure in these vessels. There is no direct pump in the body pushing lymphatic fluid. There are back-flow valves that keep lymphatic fluid moving in one direction. These lymphatic vessels are connected and travel to lymph nodes. From the lymph nodes, the swelling is eliminated from the 'interstitial space' (space around the cells) and enter back into the regular circulation.

This is a microscopic view of the **cross section** of an artery, vein, and lymphatic vessel. This is to show the relative thickness of the walls. As you can imagine the lymphatic vessels are very thin. Squeezing them too hard with a garment will cause them to collapse and not take the swelling out of your body.

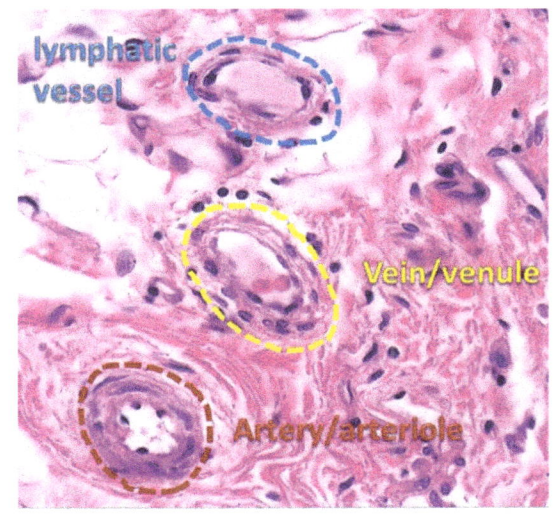

The reason this is important is because swelling is the same as lymphatic fluid that is trapped in the tissue. What does lymphatic fluid actually look like? Have you ever popped a blister? That blister is filled with clear colored lymphatic fluid. In order for the swelling to go down, it must travel from the space, down the lymphatic vessels to the lymph nodes. The areas we are typically most concerned about with swelling is the belly after liposuction 360 (lipo of the back, belly, and sides). The swelling in these areas need to eventually end up in the inguinal lymph nodes.

These nodes are located in the groin. Once in the lymph nodes it eventually drains up into the subclavian veins.

So what if the swelling is 'stuck' in your body? If swelling does not exit the area and drain the lymph nodes it can remain trapped in the area.
The body can then wall this off in the form of a seroma.
The swelling can become fibrotic and hard.
The swelling can form hard nodules, that can be visible through the skin.

So wouldn't the tightest garment be the perfect after liposuction? NO!

Imagine a giant tube of toothpaste. If you squeeze the toothpaste in the middle, the toothpaste will move from the middle to the top and the bottom of the tube. Similarly if a garment is too tight it will trap the swelling above and below the garment and not allow the swelling to drain to lymph nodes. Let me remind you again, there is no major pump pushing lymphatic fluid. And, the vessels are very weak and flimsy.

Aside from their naturally weak structure, because of the liposuction many of them are damaged or injured (a).

If the garment is compressing them, the swelling cannot travel down the vessels. The vessels will simply collapse and trap the fluid where it is (b).

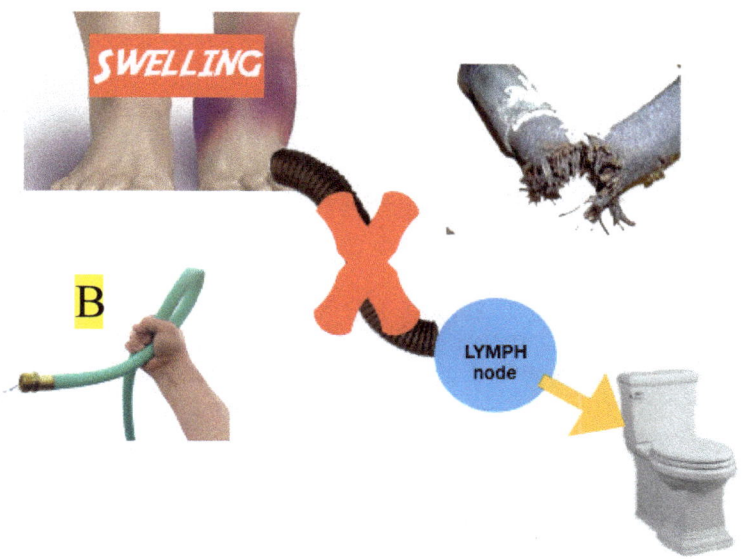

Although your friend from Colombia or the massage therapist may disagree, scientifically speaking this information is correct and should be adhered to. Dr. Klein, one of the leaders in the field of liposuction (who invented tumescent anesthesia- the technique we all use today) wrote a textbook for doctors. I include an excerpt from his book about garments here:

"Constant external compression does not increase lymphatic pumping action or facilitate lymph flow. Constant compression applied externally to the skin tends to squeeze the delicate subcutaneous lymphatic capillary, causing the lumen to collapse on itself and preventing interstitial fluid from entering. Thus excessive, continuous external compression may impede lymphatic drainage and exacerbate postoperative edema."

The Tumescent Technique, Jeffrey Klein, MD Chapter 30: Postliposuction Care: Open Drainage and Bimodal Compression.

Most people buy garments that are stock and from a catalog. This is not simply a crop top or a pair of pants. This incorporates the belly, sides, back, butt, and legs. If you haven't noticed perhaps now more than ever, people are desiring bodies that are very different than bodies of the past. Very exaggerated waist to hip ratios are more popular than ever before. It is VERY difficult to get a garment that is appropriately tight on the waste, **and** loose on the butt. Everyone has a different shape and during your recovery your shape will evolve and change and the garment you started with not not fit the same after.

After liposuction takes place, fat is removed. The skin over the body is now larger that what is necessary and the body responds by causing the skin to retract. This ability is known as the skin elasticity. This is discussed more in other chapters but bring it up here because too tight a garment will also interfere with the body's natural reaction of skin retraction. Not allowing the skin to retract and by a tight garment 'artificially putting skin where it needs to be', can create dents and furthermore can make the skin lazy. You will not get the full tightening effect that comes naturally. I have seen this most evident in the arms. For that reason I do not let my patients where any garment on their arms until a month has passed. This allows the skin to do its thing, and then once the skin settles to its new home we can help it along with some light compression. (I do place a bandage for 2 days on the arm because they leak so much fluid but this is not for compression)

Function of a garment
The garment is more for the liposuctioned areas than for the butt.

Minor point
The exception rule is a butt where fat may have shifted. I have seen post surgical patients where the fat seems to have shifted much higher than where it was intended. After seeing this at the 7 days follow up, with a few minutes of manual manipulation (me squeezing the butt), and wearing a well fitting garment, these butts ended up looking great. Do not let someone untrained to try to move the fat in your butt with manual manipulation. If you compress the area inappropriately you can pop the underlying connective tissue. And you can actually hear and feel it pop. It will hernia the fat into the skin (known as a blowout - more about that in the complications chapter) and it creates a VERY difficult problem to correct. I have seen it.

Main point
The garment is for the areas that have been liposuctioned. Its role is most important in the beginning of the postoperative period.

A research study done on brow lifts revealed that it takes 10 days to develop early attachments of the skin to the underlying tissue. It is this reason that in my opinion the first 10 days are the most important to have the skin rest in the proper position. The fat is essentially the glue between the skin and the muscle. Liposuction is a procedure that removes and breaks up that glue. After the fat is removed the skin is freely mobile and very impressionable.

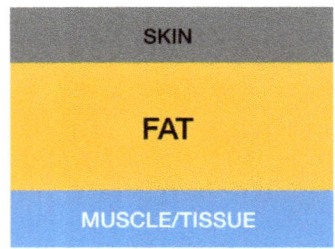 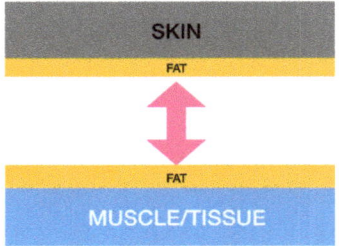

If I moved the skin to the side, and positioned it there for 10 days, it would stay there. This is why the skin after surgery needs to be in the correct position. Sitting bent over can causes indentations in the skin. Squeezing your body into a tight fitting garment will 'scrunch' your skin and crease unevenness. For that reason if I anticipate someone will have loose skin after surgery, I will have them wear a loose fitting garment. If there seems to be skin bunching i will have the patient wear a foam pad directly on the front of the belly to keep it smooth, or on the sides if the garment is creating a crease in theses areas. Some people get the firm flexible boards to place inside the garment. These are ok if creasing on the belly is noted. Foam on the sides can be helpful too if the garment is digging into the hips which can happen in patients who now have a small waist and wide hips.

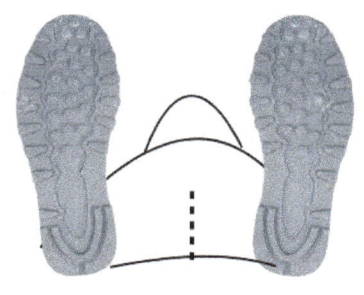
Where should the zipper be? Lets take a look at the general shape of a person from the bottom up (diagram on left). We are shaped with the middle of our body with the greatest projection outward. Therefore the greatest tightness in a tight garment is in the middle. If the zipper is there it will dig into your skin and potentially damage it. For that reason I do not like the garments with zippers in the middle.

When people sit the majority of skin bunching (right) will occur in the middle. Adding a zipper and the supporting fabric around it does not allow the garment to properly bend and flex smoothly. The zipper fabric is generally thicker and less pliable and will 'buckle' over the skin. If you are going to get a garment with a zipper it is best to get one with the zipper on the side.

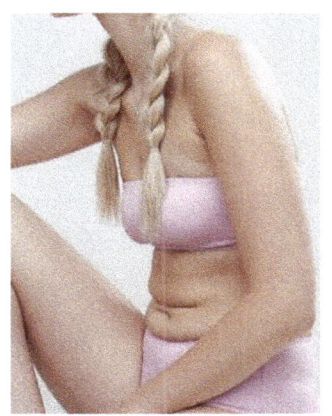

I have nothing but love for the people doing lymphatic massages and it is an important skill and part of the healing journey after this surgery. My intention here is not to belittle or insult them, but in the immediate post surgical period, I do not think it is appropriate to get advice about switching garments from anyone other than the doctor who treated you. If advice is given to you that is not in agreement with what your doctor told you, check with your doctor. For example, if the doctor does his job and does an amazing liposuction job on you. He/she then gives you a XL garment. A week later you are wearing a S garment from your massage therapist. You are not in compliance with the doctor's recommendations. If you are happy with your result, the doctor can now say you did not follow their protocol.

If you trusted your doctor enough to have surgery, trust your doctor to take care of you after. The only person that knows what happened in the operative room was your doctor.
The only one that knows how much scar tissue was under your skin was your doctor.
The only one that knows how much fat came from each area during the case was your doctor.
The only one who was under your skin and felt the thickness of your skin was your doctor.

Every patient is different and every surgery is different. Get those massages, wear your garment, but if you have a question first ask your doctor.

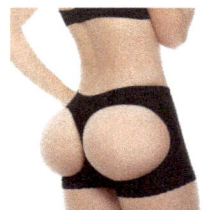

Garments like that shown here (although nice to look at) are not good for your healing after a BBL. We have had patients modify their garment like this or to cut the legs on their own because they believe it is better. This completely ruins the compression distribution. This type of garment can cause dents and cut off the circulation to the butt killing fat. It can create an undesirable shape. Garments should not be used to gross shape the butt, aside from the rare examples spoken about. It is there to support the skin after liposuction. Do not let the garment ruin hours of hard work by your doctor, and your financial investment. Talk to your doctor. If you deviate from your instructions and something comes out unsatisfactorily if becomes your fault and the doctor may wash his hands of it.

Chapter 34: Lymphatic Massages

"I got 20 freaks in my room, while I'm gettin' a massage in my room."

Future

As a medical definition, lymphedema is edema caused by inadequate lymphatic function resulting from agenesis (people born without proper lymphatics), destruction (from cancer, surgery, radiation, trauma), or obstruction (tumor compression, parasite infection etc) of lymph vessels or lymph nodes After liposuction, the lymphedema is unique in that it usually resolves spontaneously with time, typically within 2 to 6 months. Lymphatic vessels are important because they are the only vessel in the body that absorbs excessive proteins in the spaces between the cells. If these proteins are not absorbed into these cells, they will draw fluid out of surrounding areas, by the process called osmosis.

Swelling occurs when there is excessive fluid in the space outside of the cells, also known as the extracellular space. This is a result of 2 things:
    A.   Impaired lymphatic drainage
    B.   Excess filtration

We may remember from high school chemistry the theory of osmosis. Where a red blood cell was placed in an isotonic solution and it stayed the same in size. When placed in a hypertonic solution (meaning the external fluid had a higher concentration of solute) the cell would shrink.

When the cell was placed in a hypotonic solution (meaning the external fluid had a lower concentration of solute) the cell will swell. In summary this fluid follows the higher concentration of solute in an effort to dilute the solute. In the situation of liposuction the solute is proteinaceous material. Simply put, the water moves to the areas with more material (protein) to dilute it.

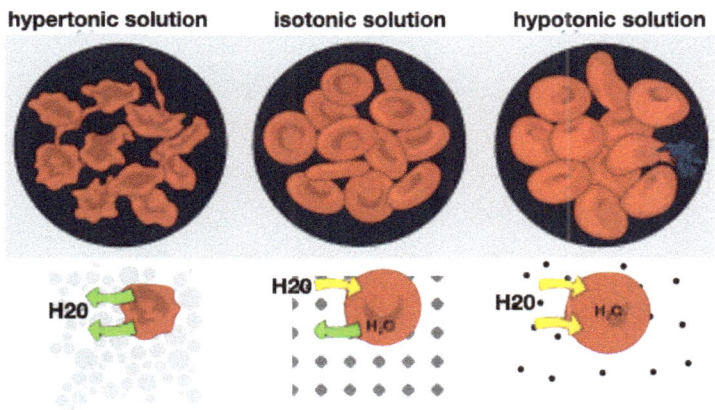

1. in the normal cell the concentration of protein materials is the same in the cell and outside the cell (isotonic)
2. hypotonic solution has more proteins inside the cell so the fluid around the cell is drawn in to normalize the balance
3. hypertonic solution has more protein outside the cell so the fluid from the cell leaves the cell (shrivels up) and enters the tissue to balance the amount of

The concept is the same in post surgical swelling after liposuction but the players are different. The intravascular space acts as the red blood cell in the above experiment and the interstitial space is the environment in which the red cell sits in the above experiment. The interstitial space is another term for the space in the tissues beneath and including the skin.

Liposuction although performed through very tiny holes, is very damaging to the tissue below the skin. Lymphatic vessels are damaged, bleeding is created and many tunnels under the skin are created that act as reservoirs for swelling to sit in. Lymphatic massage is so important to less pain, a faster recovery, skin retractions and a less chance of skin irregularities (lumps, bumps, and nodules). Take a look under a tummy tuck flap of the areas that had lipo versus the areas that did not (below).

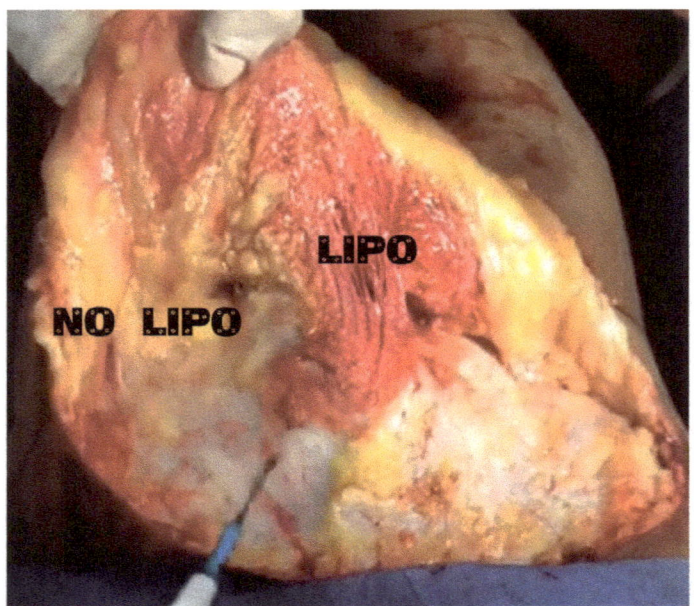

Although I have never learned it in a textbook or a medical journal, the importance of lymphatic massage after a Brazilian butt lift cannot be overstated. The post surgical lymphatic massage is very different than a traditional lymphatic massage for one that has lymphedema. Lymphedema is often seen in those after having one's lymph nodes removed during cancer surgery. In these patients, gentle strokes to the skin will encourage the stagnant lymphatic fluid to be drained. This is a different type of massage than the one after liposuction surgery.

After liposuction the patient has intact lymph nodes. Some of the fluid is lymphatic fluid from edema, and early on it is tumescent fluid that was infiltrated along with some blood. The lymphatic massage after surgery has been described as fairly painful, but incredibly relieving. After this massage patients immediately feel more mobile and less stiff.

These massages can be started as soon as 2-3 days after surgery, however most patients cannot tolerate the massage until one week. Many lymphatic massage therapists sell packages of 10 or 12. It is better to do frequent massages early rather than 12 spread out of a long amount of time. 2 or 3 massages a week is great, rather than 1 every 2 weeks.

If you get this massage early on, you may actually see fluid exiting the holes made from the access holes for the liposuction cannulas. This is not lymphatic fluid. **THIS IS TUMESCENT FLUID (NUMBING FLUID) MIXED**

WITH SOME BLOOD! When the tissue starts to heal and the opening to the outside world is closed up, the fluid remains in the body. After that, it will be appreciated when touching the skin. You will walk into the therapist hard and leave softer and smoother as it is mobilized and absorbed by your body.

After the initial drainage of tumescent (numbing) fluid from the liposuction holes that occurs over the first few days, fluid can collect in the body in one of two ways:

1. There can be a fluid collection under the skin such as a seroma that can be drained with a needle. A large amount of fluid should be drained with a needle. A small amount your body should be able to absorb on its own. It is my 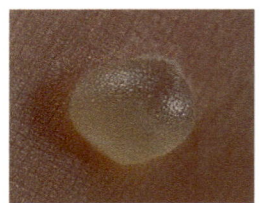 opinion that whenever possible, it should be removed. How much is a small amount? That should be left to the discretion of your doctor.

2. There could be fluid (edema aka swelling) that is soaked into the tissue (the skin) like a saturated sponge. Even if you stick a needle in a soaked sponge, nothing will come out of the needle. Instead by squeezing the sponge, the fluid is expressed. That is the purpose of these lymphatic massages. To maneuver the fluid out and to the lymph nodes.

The purpose of the lymphatic massage is the help the swelling subside quicker, allow the skin to retract better, smoothing irregularities, and nodules. By ignoring these areas of hard nodules, they can become permanently hard and fibrotic. Massage therapists like to use the word 'fibrosis' to describe this. Sometimes ignoring the need for lymphatic massages can cause a seroma that becomes encapsulated.

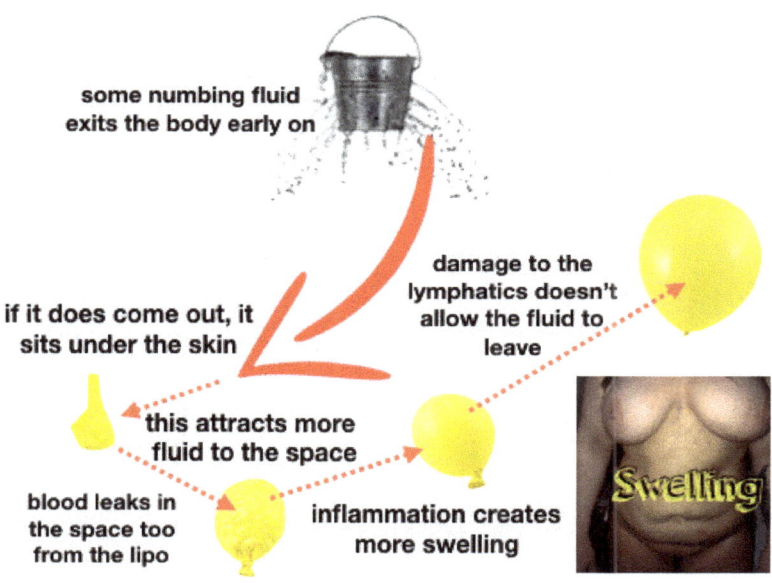

Lymphatic massage will help encourage the swelling to mobilize back into the lymphatic system some of which fluid enters the circulation while the excess liquid is sent to the kidneys and pee'd out.

As more post surgical massage places are opening and sharing their message on instagram, I wanted to make some misconceptions clear.

1. You may not have fluid pouring out of your liposuction holes during the massage. This does not mean you aren't getting a lymphatic massage. Lymphatic fluid is not the liquid coming out of your lipo holes after surgery. That is tumescent fluid and some blood from the procedure.

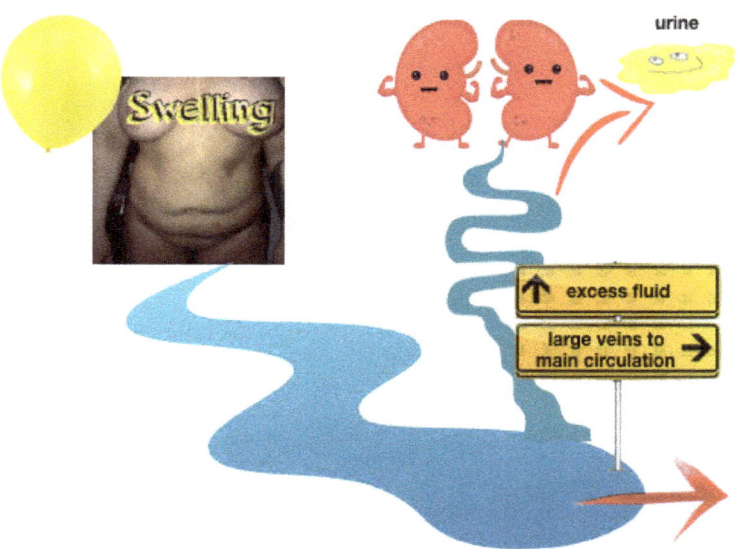

If the massage facility drains yellowish clear fluid from your liposuctioned areas, that is not lymphatic fluid. That is a seroma. If this doesn't happen that doesn't mean you didn't get a lymphatic massage. THIS A SERIOUS PET PEEVE OF MINE!!!! Patients are seeing seromas being drained by massage places and the patients are then upset to get a massage and not see the same fluid coming out during their massage. This is not because you did not get a good massage. This is not because the doctor did something wrong. This is not because your incisions were too tightly closed. This is not because you are wearing the wrong garment. The fluid that you are seeing coming out is seroma. It is a minor complication after liposuction not lymphatic fluid existing your body. It is important to get the seroma out but has nothing to do with lymphatic massage.

3. Please listen to your doctors advice with garments. It is not fair to generalize all lymphatic massage therapists but I will say many of the places our patients go return for a follow up wearing garments that are inappropriate for the surgery. They usually are much too tight. The last chapter was dedicated to garments, if you missed it.

"When interstitial pressure exceeds 1 or 2 mm Hg, the lymph flow rate reaches a plateau. Lymph flow fails to increase with higher interstitial fluid pressures, probably because of excessive tissue pressure compressing the outside area of larger lymphatic vessels, thereby impeding lymph flow. Therefore a high-compression postoperative garment is unlikely to increase the rate of lymph flow after liposuction." Dr. Klein's liposuction textbook

So in other words, too tight a garment is collapsing the lymphatic vessels and stopping their ability to move swelling out.

4. To my knowledge there is not good medical studies supporting carboxy therapy as a helpful or harmful procedure in the healing process after lipo 360/BBL. Antecdoctally, some of my patients believe it has helped them, while others didn't see any difference. I have been told it is painful. I think it may help in areas that are "stuck down" after lipo- most notably the arms.

5. Whether you use a wood stick, suction cup, hands, or a slice of pizza to massage your body, it is the mechanics of the massage, the pressure and direction of the massage that is most important. I do not believe there is a huge benefit for one thing over another.

6. Red light therapy does have some medical literature that demonstrates improved healing after surgery. It is hard to believe something works if you feel nothing from it. I do not have personal experience with it aside from our Zerona machine which was used for fat reduction. It now is used primarily as a coat hanger in my closet. Red lights on the proper wavelength however supposedly can help you heal faster. There are different wavelengths for fat reduction, pain, hair growth, digestion, amongst other applications. There are other color lights too for other purposes, such as a blue for acne.

Chapter 35: Pain

"If you want the rainbow, you gotta put up with the rain."
Dolly Parton

Pain is very subjective. We all know someone who is a major drama queen over the smallest injury (it is probably a guy). We also know the one person who can have a limb hanging on by a thread and be totally fine. It's ironic too because most people who complain the most say they have a high tolerance of pain and multiple tattoos.

This procedure hurts. We do have the occasional patient who says it was a piece of cake but the majority of patients who have lipo 360 say it is pretty bad. The discomfort doesn't come from butt injections itself, it comes from the liposuction. To add to the aggravation, you are dizzy, light headed, incredibly messy (leaking fluids) and you cant get comfortable because you cannot sit on your butt. If you are ready for it, it becomes easier. When this procedure is sensationalized as easy, and the pain comes as a surprise it makes things worse.

The pain medication you will be given will take the edge off but ***it will not take all the pain away***. The more narcotic pain medication you take the more likely you will feel nausea. The more you take it the more likely you will be constipated. Now imagine being constipated, not being able to sit on the toilet properly, and wearing a filthy tight garment that you keep having to take off and on to TRY to poop. Ahhhh, the joys of making ourselves beautiful.

We surveyed 100 patients after their lipo 360/BBL surgery and they rated their pain at its worst on the average a 9 out of 10.

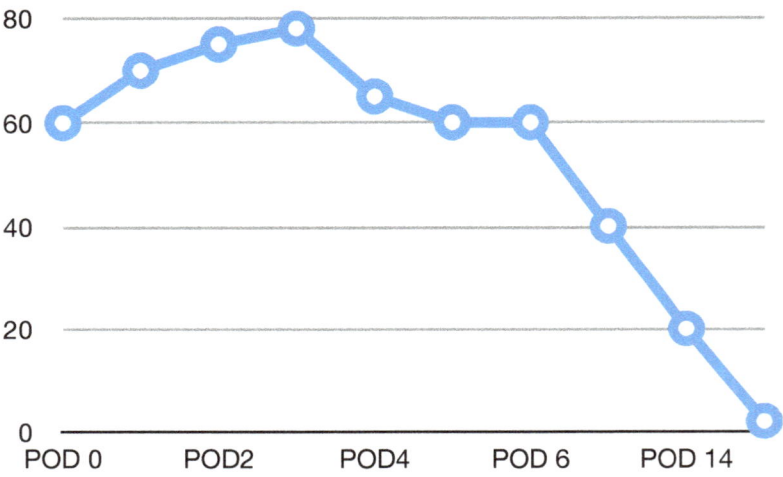

This is the distribution of pain intensity over PODs (post operative days).

Different doctors manage pain differently. The medically community as a whole are making an effort to decrease the amount of narcotics given to patients as narcotic abuse is becoming a growing epidemic in our country. For that reason, some doctors are trying to avoid giving narcotics after surgery.

CBD oil is becoming a popular supplement for pain management but there has not been any scientific data demonstrating its efficacy in this procedure.

Here is some other useful information from the survey I did from my patients.
The best way to treat pain is called pre-emptive anesthesia.

What was the worst part of your surgery (100 were asked at 1 month after lipo 360/BBL in my office)	
getting in a comfortable position	35
pain	16
massages	9
day 2	9
leaking fluid	6
constipation	6
getting our of bed	6
day 1	6
it was easy	3
1st week	3
anxiety	1

This requires three things to happen:
1. Pain meds are given to the patient **before** the first injury
2. Pain meds are given **before** the patient experiences pain.
3. Pain meds are given **before** the pain medications wear off.

Imagine your hand in luke warm water. It feels ok and your hand can stay in it. As the temperature rises, eventually you will reach a point when it is too hot and you want to take your hand out. That point of discomfort perceived as pain, lets refer to the as the "tipping point" shown below on the graph. Once your body is at or beyond that point, it is difficult to get back into a comfortable range. That is how pain works. Once you reach a "tipping point", it is hard to manage the pain.

By taking pain medications before the injury happens, will move the "tipping point" over to give you more of a

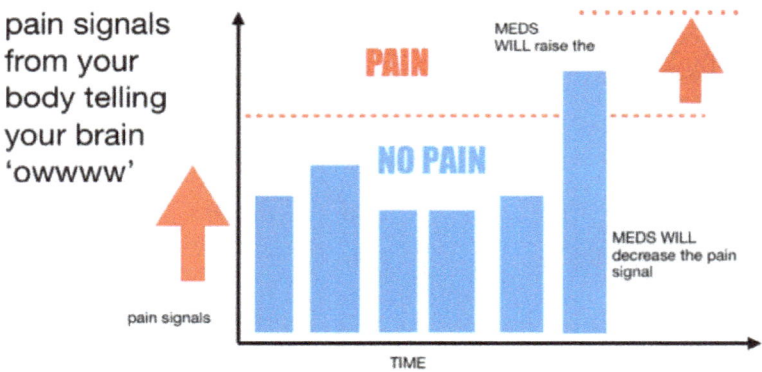

tolerance before pain is felt. Once you are past that point it is difficult to push below it again.

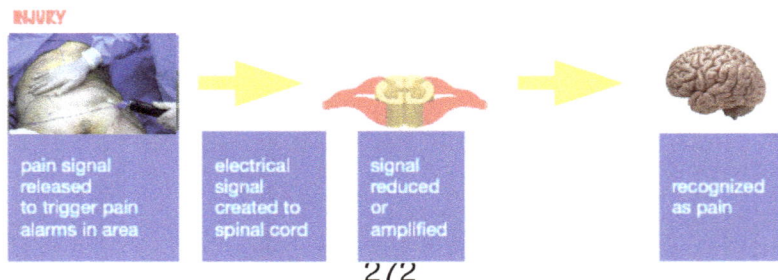

To simplify the process *(flow chart see below)*:
Pain can be stopped anywhere along this transmission process.

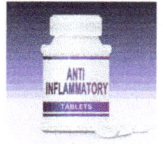
like Aspirin, Tylenol, Prednisone, Decadron, Toradol, Advil, Motrin
(stops the pain receivers from creating the starting signal)

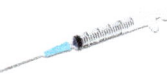
like lidocaine (in tumescent anesthesia fluid), marcaine, experil
(blocks the transmission to the spinal cord)

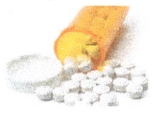
like Percocet, Vicodin, Dilaudid, Morphine, Fentanyl
(works at the level of the brain and spinal cord)

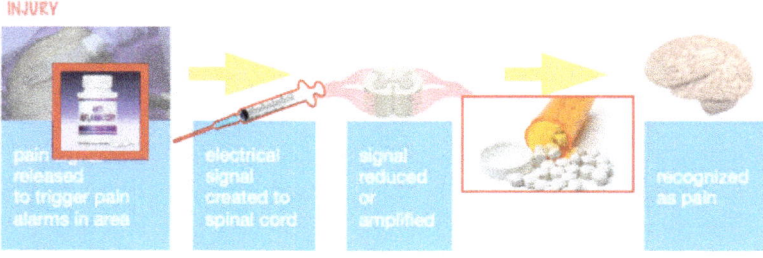

What steps can be taken to minimize pain after surgery:
1. Making sure your doctor will be doing their part to prevent the pain. Many doctors don't use local anesthesia during general anesthesia because you are not responding to the pain so they do not believe it is necessary.

Even though you are not moving, your body is still sensing the pain and will still be releasing chemicals to send the pain signal that will catch up with you later, in a bad way.

2. Make sure you have a competent anesthesia provider doing their part to control pain. For example, when you are sleeping during general anesthesia, again, you do sense pain although you not moving in response to the pain. The pain you are feeling will show in an increase in heart rate. Pain medication will bring this heart rate back to normal. So will certain blood pressure meds (which have nothing to do with pain management). So instead of addressing the cause of the increased heart beat, your anesthesia provider could potentially treat the symptom of an increased heart beat ignoring the fact that you may be experiencing pain.

3. YOU should take some type of pain medication even if you are not in pain for the first 3 days or so. Over the counter meds can be taken but some cannot be taken in conjunction with narcotics. For example, Percocet is [Acetaminophen + hydrocodone]. Tylenol is [acetaminophen]. If you take Percocet and 2 hours later take Tylenol, you can overdose because they both share the ingredient of acetaminophen.

Ask your doctor if you can supplement Ibuprofen between narcotic doses if you are still so uncomfortable. I often recommend for example: take 2 Percocets at 12:00, 2 Advils at 2:00, 2 Percocets at 4:00, 2 Advils at 6:00.

After surgery, some people complaining of itching or electric shocks. Often patients get relief after taking Benadryl or Allegra. Please check with your doctor before doing so. This is usually a normal reaction of the nerves healing after surgery. If it is very uncomfortable, your doctor may prescribe Gabapentin (Neurontin).

In summary, the pain from a BBL/lipo 360 for most is difficult.

- Staying ahead of the pain will help.
- Moving around will help. People tend to get stiff when not moving enough.
- Lymphatic massages will help the pain go away quicker.
- When you take a shower, put your faja in the freezer. When you put a cool faja (garment) back on it will provide some relief.
- Make sure you talk to your doctor before taking *any* medication.

The pain meds will help with some relief but do not expect total relief from the medications.

Chapter 36: More patient feedback

At what times did you feel at your most comfortable?

I asked 100 of my BBL patients at their 1 month follow up this question. Here are the real results:

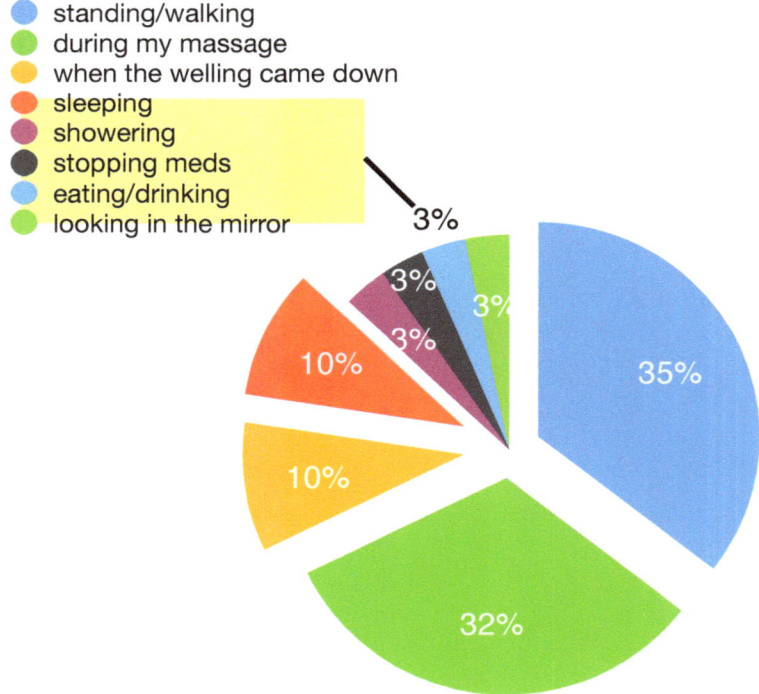

Chapter 37: Exercising

"If you are in a bad mood go for a walk. If you are still in a bad mood go for another walk."
Hippocrates

The short end of the story is after 8 weeks there are no restrictions for exercise. I do recommend some exercise leading up to this 8 week landmark.

Fat is the glue that attaches the skin to the underlying tissues. I reference this statement many times throughout this book. During liposuction that glue is disrupted and the skin is freely mobile. It takes 10 days for the skin to form an early attachment to the tissue. For the first 2 weeks we want to make sure the skin is flat and in the right position on the belly.

Week 1
During this period you are recovering from a major assault on your body. Exercise should not be done at all. In fact not much should be done at all aside from resting, eating, showering, going to the bathroom. It is a good idea to walk around out of bed but no exercising.

Week 2
At this point it is ok to do some more walking around your house and it is encouraged. Lymphatic vessels are stimulated (as are your bowels) by movement. As the

muscles in your body help you move, the lymphatic vessels are helped along to eliminate swelling.

After this week as mentioned above, the skin has started to form a union with the tissue beneath it. This early adhesion can be overpowered by too much movement. I had a patient driving her car and reached to the back seat to get something and she felt a pop. Sure enough she 'broke' this early attachment. In this space she developed a seroma. This did not alter her final result but was a more of a nuisance to manage. I ask my patients to move like a robot. To bend at the knees if they need something low. To use a step stool rather than reach to get something from the top shelf. If you need something from the back seat of the car, get out and walk to the back seat.

Week 4
Some light treadmill work is ok. Be sure to be wearing your faja and listen to your body. If it doesn't feel right, don't do it. I would not do much more than a brisk walk, maybe 4 mph or less.

Week 6
At this point exercise is a good idea. Arms, shoulders, chest, legs, abs, back are all fair game. I would not perform anything that uses the glutes. The stem cells in butt are still growing and lactic acid in the muscles, and tightening the glutes as a working muscle I believe can negatively affect the fat. I would not recommend squats, deadlifts, or lunges until the 8 week mark. This is my opinion.

<u>8 weeks and beyond</u>
Exercise is wonderful and will only enhance your butt shape. It can add more muscle and raise the butt up. It **will not** create any roundness to the sides of the butt.

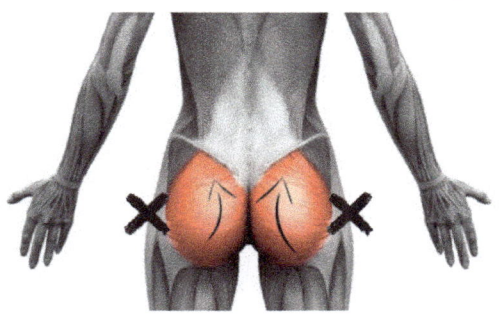

Chapter 38: Incisions and secret tips

"Please don't cut me off, know you got the sauce."
Tory Lanez

<u>Mr. Softy and the evening before surgery</u>

Yes, it may be a while before you can have sex but I'm not referring to that. I am referring to a trick I was taught from one of my mentors while training in Texas. This old timer had incredible results from liposuction. This was before the time of aggressive liposuction that we do today[3]. His results were so good that his colleagues accused him of 'doctoring' (photoshopping) his before and after pictures. He was brought before the board and he actually presented Polaroids of his pictures to the board proving they were this actual results and the case was dismissed. After building a friendship with him, he told me the secret to his great results for liposuction was Blue Bonnet Ice Cream.

The night before surgery he would instruct his patients to binge on ice cream. For very skinny people, start a few days before surgery. If I fear we may be a little low on fat for a fat transfer I now instruct the same. I am not sure if Blue Bonnet ice cream is readily available but I would go all in with regular ice cream that has a high fat content. This is not the time to get calorie conscience with non fat

---

[3] When I was taught liposuction I was taught to leave a protective layer of fat underneath the skin. This gives a more natural look and feel to the skin. While it is still acceptable to do such a thing, most of the patients seeking out liposuction nowadays want more extreme results and this protective layer of fat is no longer left behind.

frozen yogurt. If you have enough fat this step is not necessary.

The rationale behind this is simple. After puberty barring some extreme gain in weight, we do not grow more fat cells. The fat cells that we have are the fat cells that we die with (assuming they are not surgically removed). Those limited fat cells can however grow in size. It was the belief of this surgeon that the fat cells transiently 'bloat up' soon after eating this high caloric food, thus making it easier to remove during liposuction. I am unaware of any scientific literature supporting this, just anecdotal experience. I will say I have seen what appears to look like a nice yellow fat come out. One would have to suck out the fat of the same person and the same area with the same technique before and after ice cream to really know if it works, but there is no harm in eating that extra ice cream and through personal experience, I will attest to some benefit. And no one can argue, ice cream is lit.

Please do not take this as medical advice. Particularly if you have diabetes, have a BMI greater than 32 or lactose intolerant. We certainly don't want you to have diarrhea all over the operating room table the next day.
No one wins there.

The deal with lipo foam or boards

For those who have no idea what I am talking about here are some pictures:

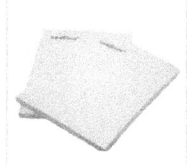	This is referred to as lipofoam and is often placed under the garment for what many believe adds needed extra compression

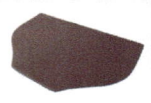	This is referred to as an abdominal board which goes under the garment.
	This is a firm foam with a harder piece inside that goes between your skin and the garment. It is placed on the back with the point going down the lower back.
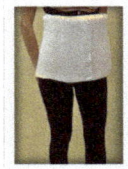	This is a full body soft foam wrap that is sometimes placed in addition to the traditional garment after surgery.

Is foam or a board necessary on everyone? No. Is there a role for foam or a board in the right situation? Absolutely! So here is the deal:

AFTER LIPOSUCTION 360

For a patient with thick skin using foam can help but certainly won't hurt. Feel free to check out Chapter 4 on skin thickness if you missed it. What the foam can be used for is:

1. Many times the garment will create folds or indentations in the skin. These can be quite evident in a thin skinned person. The foam should be used between the skin and the garment in the indentation. Sometimes this happens where the zipper is. Check out 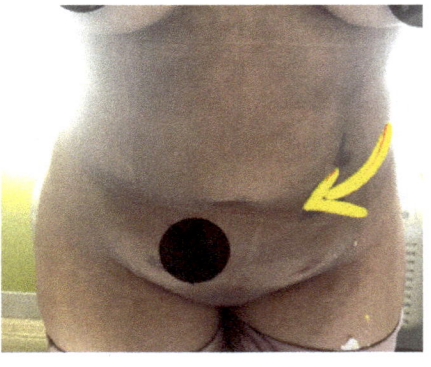 Chapter 33 about garments. Often the indentations are

seen across the belly sometimes on the sides. The foam should go where the indent is. After 10 days of this indent staying without any intervention, I fear the indentation can potentially stay there.

2. For someone who has a lot of loose skin the foam can be quite helpful. These are people who probably would have benefited from a tummy tuck but for one reason or another s getting liposuction only. For these people the skin will often naturally fold right above the pubis area.

As described in multiple other chapters, fat is the glue that attaches the skin to the underlying tissue. After the fat is removed and interrupted from liposuction, after 10 days the skin begins its reattachment. If the excess skin is allow to fold down in these patients with extra loose skin, the fold will become a permanent one. In 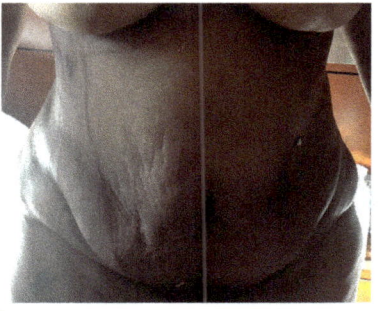 these patients I recommend once their garment is on, to pull the skin up towards their breasts and place a piece of foam to hold the skin up. Much like a woman pulling her breasts up in a bra.

3. For those patients whom happen to develop a seroma, after it is drained it is important to keep extra pressure on this potential space where the fluid was just drained from. This can prevent the seroma from filling up again. A piece of foam over the spot can add some localized pressure to the spot and help prevent the seroma from recurring or at least minimizing the size of it.

4. Foam on the lower back is important for a few reasons, especially after a lipo 360/BBL. I personally have very few patient with a seroma in this area, but my colleagues tell me they do all the time. Some of that is liposuction technique and it may also be because of the foam we place in the spot. This is an area where we want absolute adherence of the skin down to the bone. Keep the foam in this spot will help the skin stay down. We leave our foam on for 10 days. As explained in other sections of this book, that is time it takes for the skin to start to stay down. Additionally, having a butt full to capacity with fat and a back that has been sucked out and is essentially empty makes for potential avalanche. All the areas under the skin are connected. All of that pressure in your butt can potentially shoot all the fat into the hollow space where all the fat has been removed if too much pressure is applied externally to the butt. Too tight a garment, sitting too early, or sitting incorrectly can all send the fat into the back. The foam acts as a mechanical barrier to keep the fat down. It also serves to hold the skin down to allow it to stick. And lastly, it mentally is a reminder to avoid putting pressure on your butt.

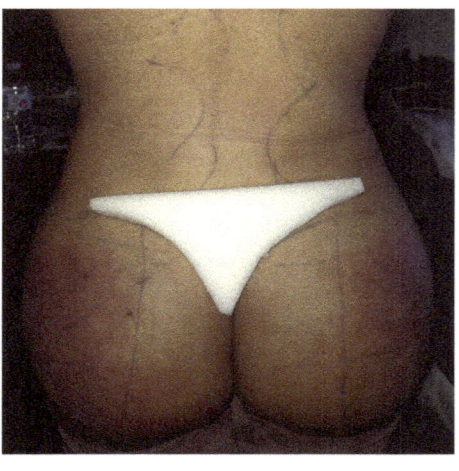

Imagine injecting a blue dye under the skin at the level of the shoulder blades. Let's pretend this stain does not get absorbed by any cells/tissue along the way. Eventually this blue dye would make it down to the feet. This example is to

demonstrate how every part of the body is connected in layers, much like a sandwich.

AFTER A TUMMY TUCK AND A BBL TOGETHER

Foam can be quite helpful after this combination and a hard board can be used but one must be VERY careful using it on the tummy tuck. If you are using a traditional binder and you have a medium to large size butt with nice hips, you will probably hate this binder. The struggle is, it will continuously hit your hips and slide up on the sides. It will result in a position that is too high for the tummy and sit too far above the scar. It will also bunch quite a bit on the sides that will annoy and irritate the skin on the sides.

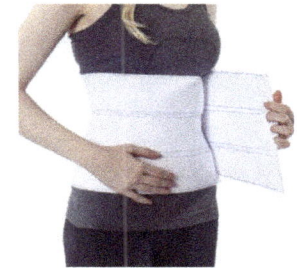

After a tummy tuck the skin is often numb and you may not even realize the garment is doing damage to your skin. Almost always when using a binder after a tummy tuck it is a good idea to have foam on the sides of the binder. An alternative is the aforementioned foam wrap demonstrated in the bottom photo of the prior chart.

A hard ab board with a binder can be used as long as the board is being used in the midline, to ease the transition from no binder to binder. It can be used as an extension of your binder. Placing the board on the top part of the binder, for those with a long torso, will allow for compression where the garment cannot reach. Similarly, it can be placed below the incision line on the bottom if you are 'puffy' there. It is very important to make the edges of the board do not dig in to the incision. Again, you may not

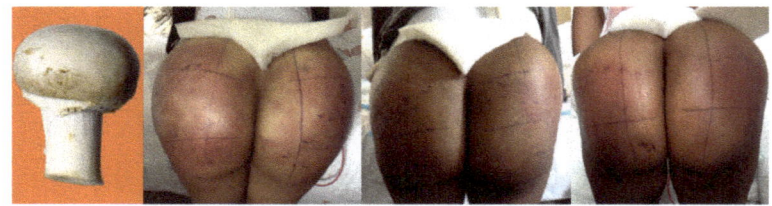

have complete feeling at this point of healing and may not realize you are damaging the skin.

An odd phenomenon can often happen to the butt when a BBL and a tummy tuck area done at the same time. The fat will often sneak up a little; mixed with swelling, can give the butt a very odd appearance. It is usually from the garment or binder being very tight around the waist with little to no pressure on the butt. Patients will often get freaked out and I don't blame them for it. It will look like a mushroom ass. This is the one time I like massages on the top part of the butt. It usually will normalize with time (a week or two). For this reason If I fear this may happen with my patient I will put foams a little more on the sides than I normally do and under fill the top portion of the butt expecting some migration upward of fat, as demonstrated in the photos.

PLACEMENT OF THE ENTRY POINT HOLES

The holes made for liposuction are generally quite small. The cannulas diameter used are usually 4-5 mm for large areas like the belly back and sides. If one were going to perform liposuction on smaller areas such as the knees or neck a smaller cannula is often used and the holes are smaller. The holes made are usually a little larger than the cannula diameter. It is sometimes better to have a hole a little bigger to limit the friction from the cannula. *That's what she said.* But is is true. A larger hole will heal better than a small hole that has been beaten up with too much friction.

Ultrasonic lipo (like Vaser lipo) uses a plastic protective piece that is temporarily sewn into the hole. The cannula is then placed inside the sleeve. This is because the ultrasonic cannula gets quite hot and can burn the skin. The downside is, in my opinion, the hole is quite large.

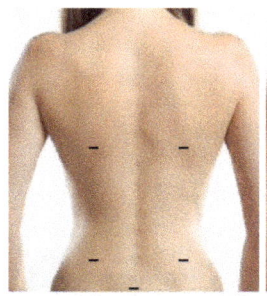

some place symmetric hidden audits (holes)

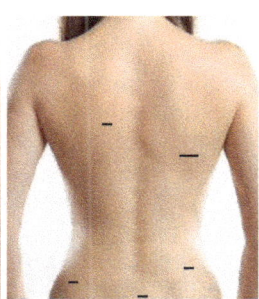

some purposely place asymmetric hidden audits (holes)

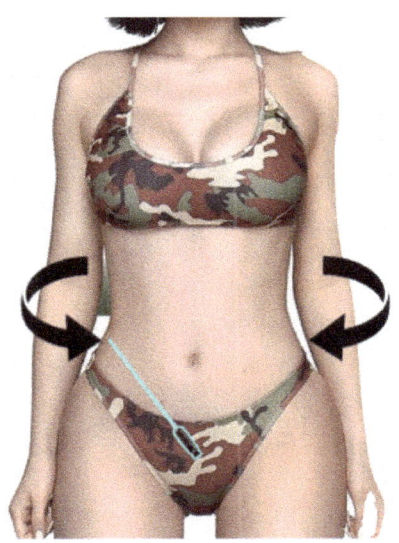

Holes are made with a scalpel blade or an audit (small tissue punch). Regardless of what is used ideally the holes should be hidden. They can be hidden in the belly button, under the underwear, or bra, in a tattoo, or in an existing scar. There are some doctors who believe holes that are made asymmetrically on purpose are less obvious than holes that are made in the same spot on both sides.

The number of liposuction holes for lipo of the abdomen for my patients are 3. 1 inside the upper belly button and 2 along the lower underwear line. If there is a tattoo or scar already there I will try to use that. If someone has a prominent rib cage and i believe there is an above average risk of potentially sliding the cannula accidentally under the rib cage, I make an additional small access hole high under the breast fold. If someone has another isolated fat pocket ,another incision made be needed near it. There are patients who want abdominal etching done. This is when the fat is removed to give the appearance of a 6 pack. Sometimes additional small incisions are needed to chisel out the ab muscles. The challenge for the surgeon is the body has curves to it and it is not a straight box. The cannulas used are straight so in order to negotiated the curves around the waist, the hole position should be in a position that is easy to go around the hip bone, and can allow the doctor to properly snatch the waist.

From those three holes, the entire abdomen and part of the flanks are suctioned. It is suctioned in a fanning technique as demonstrated in the adjacent photo. Some physicians prefer not to limit themselves to three holes in

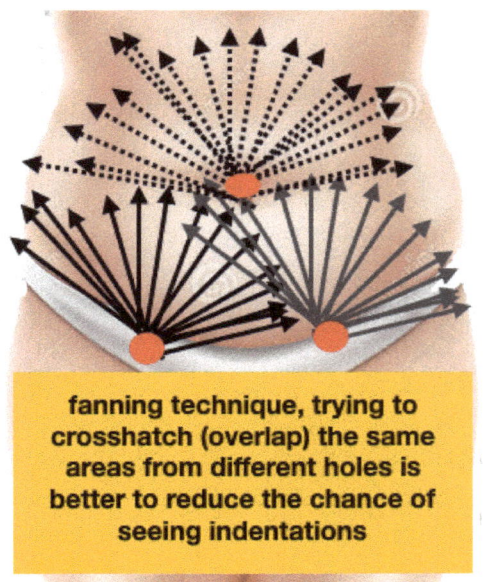

fanning technique, trying to crosshatch (overlap) the same areas from different holes is better to reduce the chance of seeing indentations

fear that the constant suction originating from those points will result in cannula indentations as seen on this celebrity photo. These are more noticeable on thin skinned patients which is covered elsewhere in this book.

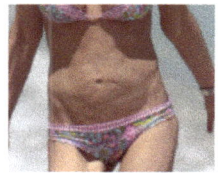

The holes on the back are generally one or two for the upper back, and three on the lower back. These are

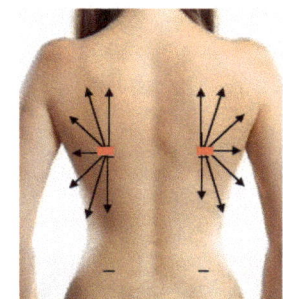

2 upper access holes
(used for 150 strokes each)
2 scars with less friction

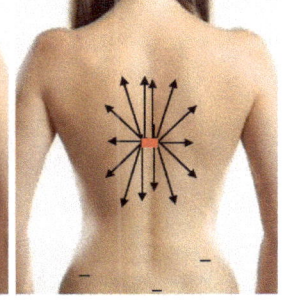

1 upper access hole
(used for 300 strokes)
1 scar with more friction

demonstrated in the below photo. I prefer to make two holes on the upper back that are hidden under the bra-line. There are some doctors that chose one in the midline. My thinking is for the same reasons mentioned above. The cannula is straight I do not think one can appropriately get around to the side of the back without having a hole that is not in the midline. Also, with two holes you are now dividing the amount of liposuction strokes and friction by two. The one hole in the middle I believe will be abused by stretching it too much, and suctioning both side through the one hole will damage the skin too much.

The lower back usually has two incisions on the peak of the butt that is used for suctioning the back and injecting the butt. There is also one in the middle of the lower back, in the but crease, used for the same. The other incisions are in the lower butt crease under the butt which are used for fat injection.

The incision for the fat injections under the butt are actually an important but overlooked thought. If you have a square butt along the bottom the incision placement can help round it out. This is one of my own secrets that I'm not sharing. I got too many doctors out there trying to cop my style.

SHOULD THE HOLES BE SEWN CLOSED OR LEFT OPEN?

So all holes from this procedure can either be left open or sutured closed. The sutures can be permanent or dissolvable, if permanent sutures are used, they should be removed after a week. In a perfect world the lipo holes on the belly especially those in a gravity dependent area (lower incisions) should be kept open. This will allow the fluid injected inside to drain, allow bleeding to exit, and may help prevent seromas. I do think if the fluid comes out sooner, the recovery is faster and people can see their results quicker. The downside of keeping them open is the scarring may be worse, people get freaked out seeing all the fluid coming out, and it may prolong bleeding. If left open, they usually start to close in the first 3 days or so.

Lipo holes sutured closed	Lipo holes left open
scar is better	drains better
bleed loss is less	less chance of seroma
less scary to see all the 'pink liquid' coming out	heals quicker to reach the endpoint of swelling

Lipo holes sutured closed	Lipo holes left open
less messy	

On the upper back I believe the holes should be closed. Typically there is not much drainage from these holes because gravity brings the fluid to the bottom.

On the lower back and butt, these holes should be closed to prevent the fat from coming out.

So in summary, in my practice, the back is completely sutured closed. The abdomen I place one suture that is a little loose to guide the skin in the correct direction and still allow for fluid to come out. I may suture the holes tight if I think the the patient or family taking care of the patient are 'worriers' or squeamish, or if they had a low hemoglobin and are oozing more than usual. If I were getting lipo on myself, I would keep my holes open but in fear of keloiding patients (whom I get a lot of) or patients super concerned about scarring, I compromise with 1 loose stitch on each hole on the front.

Chapter 39: What do I put on my scars?

"I find flaws attractive. I find scars attractive."
Angelina Jolie

<u>I do not have incentive from any company listed here.</u>

Whenever a cut is made it heals with some scar. The only time a cut can be made and heal with no scar at all is a fetus while in the mother's uterus. This has lead to experimental cleft lip and cleft palate repair, and spina bifida surgery that was just performed recently for the first time done with an endoscope in the mother's uterus but I truly doubt we will ever be doing a BBL on a fetus in utero. So you will have to settle with a scar, sorry. The good news is they are small and made in hidden areas.

A scar's surface texture can heal one of three ways:

1. Normal healing. The color of a normal healed scar is usually white, flat and thin. Sometimes it is pigments either red or brown in color.
2. Over exaggerated healing falls into 2 categories often confused by patients:

    a. **Hypertrophic scars**: This is when a scar is thick and overgrown but is confined to the margins of the cut (below)

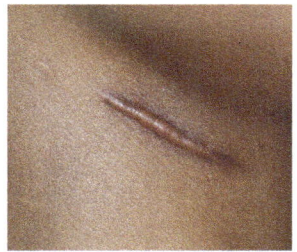

b. **Keloid scar**: This is when a scar is thick and overgrown and grows beyond the borders of the cut. **This occurs in 10% of the population.**

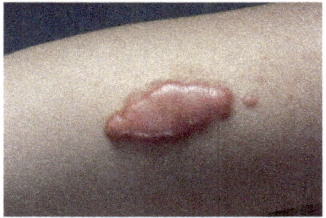

Other is factors for a keloid are darker skinned patients, Asian, Latino, being pregnant or younger than 30. If one or both of your parents had keloid scars, you are more likely also.

What do I put on my scars?

In the beginning stages of healing my preference is vaseline or aquaphore. Skin cells thrive under this medium. I ask my patients to keep this on when the sutures are still in place and until any scabbing comes off. Patients alway seem to replace this with Neosporin or Bacitracin. These ointments are good on dirty wounds but are not my preference in surgical wounds. Vitamin E is often placed on the scars also, but this should not be placed on fresh wounds. Vitamin E is good for old scars (1 year old or more).

Silicone scar treatment is clinically proven to be effective, easy to use, and low risk. Silicone is made from combining silicon and oxygen atoms. It creates a protective barrier over a scar to help the scar retain moisture. Basically, silicone is an extremely powerful moisturizer.

Steroid Injections for Hypertrophic and Keloid Scars:
Steroid injections inhibits fibroblast growth, reducing the amount of collagen deposited into the scar, and have thus been a mainstay in therapy for keloids and hypertrophic scars. Potential side 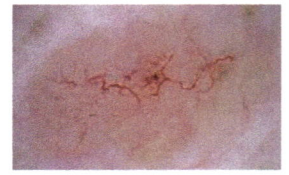 effects include hypopigmentation (less than normal pigmentation compared to the surrounding skin), atrophy, and telangiectasias (small dilated blood vessels near the surface of the skin-photo). Studies have shown that scar recurrence is common but steroid injection is generally considered effective for reduction of hypertrophic and keloid scars. Other injections include 5 Fluorouracil (5 FU) which is nice in that it will not cause skin thinning as a steroid can, or bleomycin. I often inject 5 FU and Kenalog together.

<u>**Mederma® Scar Gel**</u> – Mederma® claims to be the "#1 doctor-recommended" product for scars. It contains a

proprietary botanical extract made from onion and allantoin.

Bio-Oil – This is a popular scar treatment product that's formulated with plant extracts and vitamins suspended in an oil base. Its primary ingredients are oils of calendula, lavender*, rosemary and chamomile, along with vitamins A and E. Bio-Oil also includes fragrance and artificial color. Also consider: 1) The basic ingredient is mineral oil, a low quality oil that can not only ruin your shirts, but is also <u>linked to cancer</u>. 2) The studies proving its effectiveness are <u>misleading and incomplete</u>. 3) There's <u>not one significant ingredient</u> proven to improve scars that can't be found in numerous other products for less money. But hey, some people love it.

Arnica Cream or Gel: Applied topically, Arnica creams and gels are used to relieve pain and inflammation and promote scar healing. Avoid gels that include alcohol, which has a drying effect on skin — the opposite of what you want to do to scar tissue. You can sometimes find topical arnica formulated with calendula and silicone, both of which can also improve scar healing. Arnica is excellent at decreasing bruising.

Laser Scar Removal and Revision: Laser technology offers promising treatment for the cosmetic and functional improvement of scars, including <u>laser assisted scar healing (LASH)</u> and Pulsed Dye Laser. Fractional laser technology delivers rapid, reliable scar revision and removal and is associated with less risk, pain and downtime compared to surgical solutions. Microneedling is another option that has a similar effect as a fractional laser that is usually less expensive

If a patient is unhappy with the color of the scar I will push my finger on it and pull it away. If it turns white upon pressure and then the color returns, this is a sign of a hyperemic scar (more blood vessels growing in the scar). These many times will simply fade with time, and often progressively gets redder until the 8th week. Intense pulse light or Broad band light can help make the redness go away quicker for these types of scars. Theses are treatments with a laser, done by a spa or doctor's office.

If they do not blanch with pressure it is more of a stain in the skin. There are specific lasers for different pigments but lightening creams may work. Hydroquinone is a common lightening cream and can be costly and usually is not covered any insurance (what else is new). Be careful if you are using this. It can lighten the skin around it accidentally. Use a small amount and clean your hands after applying it. Closely monitor the results to not overshoot. There are milder lightening creams that are more cost effective such as DrBfixin's Booty Box Cream. It is available on cameosurgery.com in the online store.

Massaging the scars for 30 seconds or so a few times a day will also improve the appearance and make the scar softer.

The summary of scar management is the scars should always be hydrated and out of the sun for 9 months after the incision is made. Silicone is a great moisturizer. Some of my patients have used silicone strips which are great in that it is 24/7 moisture locked but have gotten reactions from the adhesive on the strip that look worse than the scar.

My two go to topicals are:
Scarguard MD®: It comes as almost a nail polish that is painted on the wounds. It's nice that it won't ruin your clothes and its kinda fun to pull it off when its time to reapply it It's main ingredients include **Silicone** (12%), Hydrocortisone (0.5%).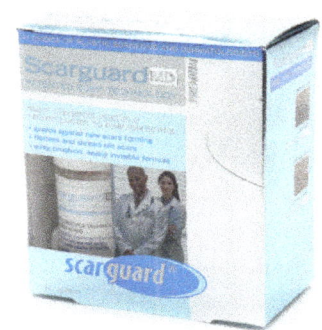
Two excellent ingredients to any scar cream.

My Spanish patients love **Cicatricure**®. The ingredients include Water, Glycerin, Carbomer, Propylene Glycol, Chamomilla Recutita (Matricaria) Flower Extract, Allium Cepa (Onion) Bulb Extract, Polysorbate 20, Phenoxyethanol, Centella Asiatica Extract, DMDM Hydantoin, Sodium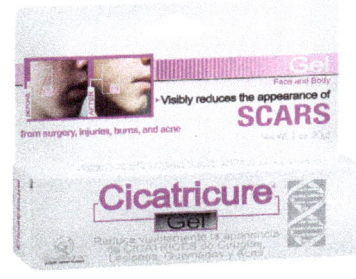
Hydroxide, Aloe Barbadensis Leaf Extract, Diazolidinyl Urea, Sodium Benzoate, Disodium EDTA, Allantoin, Citrus

Aurantium Bergamia (Bergamot) Fruit Oil, Phytonadione. You may notice Silicone is not in the ingredients. I agree. But you know, sometimes its hard to argue with Spanish women! lol (that was a joke, take it easy everyone)

If a wound is starting to look a little rough. Not infected, but just beaten up. This can be from the garment irritating the scab or just because of having super sensitive skin. This could even be from a reaction to the adhesive from your foam. I love this cream. There are some imposters making similar creams with similar names but this is the OG. It pulls off miracles. It is great for burns, and open wounds.

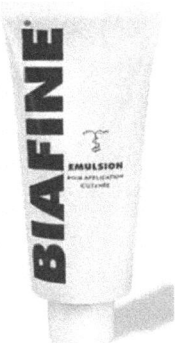

If you are prone to keloids or hypertrophic scars it is best to attack them early with steroids. Low dose radiation is an another excellent option but you would have to seek out a doctor that has such a device, as they are not commonplace in most offices.

Chapter 40: Shit people will try to sell you that's bullshit

"I'm a hustler, baby; I sell water to a well"
Jay-Z

1. PRP

PRP (platelet rich plasma) is a concentrated mixture of platelets in plasma, obtained by centrifugation of whole blood. Inside the platelets are tiny containers called alpha granules that have growth factors that promote wound healing by promoting the growth of new blood vessels and the production of tissue scaffolding. There are so many of these growth factors, most notable are names like platelet-derived growth factor, transforming growth factor-b (TGF-B), vascular endothelial growth factor (VEGF), epithelial growth factor (EGF), insulin-like growth factor, fibroblast growth factor, and platelet-derived angiogenesis factor.

Does it work to enhance your BBL result?
There are thousands of articles about PRP use however, there is no data that convincingly says it does help.
In a test tube: it shows conflicting data. Some articles shows it helps fat retention others says it hurts it
In animals: it has been shown to help
In humans: some shows it helps others show it does nothing

In my opinion, I do not think it helps as an added expense. There are some platelets being injected along with the fat in the blood. I do think there may be some benefit in decreasing pain in the butt if it is added. I have seen in my experience patients reporting less pain. I did used to inject PRP with the fat in my BBLs in thin patients who barely had enough fat for a nice booty and I was fearful that they would lose the expected 30% and not be happy afterwards. In my estimation, I do think they lost less fat than many of my other patients. However, I am not convinced it was from the PRP. My belief is since there was a scarcity of fat to begin with, after the butt was filled, it was not very tight. I think that was a factor in helping improve the blood supply and retention of the fat injected.

Does PRP cause a 'butt lift' alone, like it is advertised in some places? **Absolutely not.** It may look a touch bigger because of the sheer volume of PRP injected but as the PRP is absorbed by the body (a day or two later), the butt will look as it did before the PRP injection. Please do not go somewhere for PRP injections into the butt to get a larger butt without fat. It may help the skin quality a little but that's it.

2. HBO

This refers to hyperbaric oxygen (HBO) therapy, where the patient breathes air that contains 100 percent oxygen. (Room air contains 21 percent oxygen.) You'll have hyperbaric oxygen therapy inside a special pressurized chamber, allowing your lungs to absorb greater amounts of oxygen as you breathe.

HBO has been shown to be effective in treating;
- decompression sickness
- an air or gas embolism
- anemia due to severe blood loss
- some brain and sinus infections

- carbon monoxide poisoning
- burns resulting from heat or fire
- skin grafts
- necrotizing soft tissue infections
- osteomyelitis, a bone marrow infection
- arterial insufficiency, or low blood flow in the arteries
- acute traumatic ischemia, which may involve a crush injury, for example

gas gangrene
- a radiation injury, for example, as a result of cancer treatment

There are undoubtedly some benefits in in the treatment but what about for a BBL?

So there are two issues with this:
A. The machines that doctors are advertising to be giving hyperbaric oxygen therapy, are they actually giving hyperbaric oxygen therapy
B. If they are giving hyperbaric oxygen therapy (**Spoiler alert** they are not), does hyperbaric oxygen even help maintain the fat transfer better than without out?

To address Part A:

There are three types of hyperbaric oxygen chamber

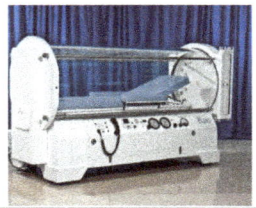
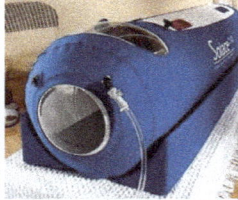

Monoplace Hyperbaric Chambers
a single patient breathes 100% oxygen while monitored multiplace hyperbaric chamber, multiple patients sit or recline while being monitored breathing 100% oxygen

Multiplace

Soft hyperbaric chambers are bags made of polyurethane or canvas material. They reach a much lower pressure and only compress room air, which contains about 21% O2 vs. the 100% medical grade O2 used in a traditional

Monoplace and multiplace hyperbaric chambers are FDA-approved for 14 different conditions, and many more indications have been or are currently being, studied using these chambers.

Soft chambers, are only FDA approved for Acute Mountain Sickness and have not been FDA approved for any other condition.

Inflatable chambers can achieve internal pressures over 1.3 ATA. Scientific studies show that oxygen blocks bacterial growth at 1.5ATA and that pressures lower than this cannot kill bacteria but will actually enhance the growth of certain molds, fungus and aerobic bacteria. *So, some doctors I have approached about 'selling a treatment that doesn't work", they responded to me by telling me "well, if it doesn't help, it can't hurt", well, apparently, it can hurt.*

- *An inflatable machine will never be used in a hospital or reputable medical office because it is not FDA approved as a medical device to deliver hyperbaric oxygen*

- Inflatable bag chambers are made with rubber, plastic and petroleum products which give off-gas in oxygen environments and expose those inside of them to toxicity by inhalation.

- Normally, we breathe 21% oxygen at sea level. Approved Hyperbaric chambers can help provide 100% oxygen saturation safely and effectively. Inflatable bag chambers only provide 26%—that's only a 5% difference from what you already breathe. Soft chambers cannot double or triple your oxygen saturation like medical grade hyperbaric oxygen therapy. True hyperbaric oxygen therapy can increase your cellular oxygen by 10, 15 or 20 times the amount (or 200%), which is what is required for wound healing.

The oxygen masks (non rebreather masks) hooked up to oxygen in the doctors offices has a higher concentration of oxygen than these inflatable chambers.

ALL of the research and medical case studies that reveal positive results using HBOT are used with medical grade steel chambers and not with inflatable chambers. Still, manufacturers and those treating patient with inflatable chambers are using this research, which is misleading. They do not produce the same results.

Even if the inflatable HBO chambers did offer the same results as the hard shell medical grade ones (only available in hospitals), does it help with fat retention? It has not been shown to help. There is no such research at all in humans. In mice, it has been shown to not have any significant change in fat volume. In theory, it sounds good, but it does not work. *At this point the persons 'selling these treatments', are misinformed or just trying to trick patients into ineffective treatments.*

3. **Suction cup**s - yes, if you have day a the beach at 1 pm with your friends that you want to flex, get this done at 12 pm. But as a long term alternative to a BBL, nonsense.

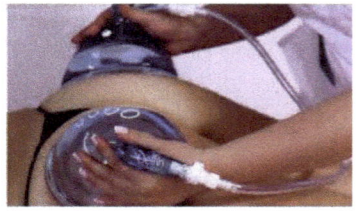

4. **Scaffolds** There are two types of scaffolds that can be added to the fat before grafting: synthetic or biologic. There has been some experimental papers showing an improvement in fat survival initially however the scaffold no not seem to disintegrate at the proper period of time for it to be useful. I have never added a scaffold to my fat and I have received samples from companies that swear their product works. It is my belief that even if instead of losing 30% of the fat transferred as we would expect, is it really worth an added expense to retain another few percent. For that reason I do not use it and do not believe it is warranted.

5. Suction cup therapy at the time of BBL with CO2 gas (carboxypneumondissection)

CO2 Pneumodissection is a technique of injecting CO2 gas under the skin during a BBL procedure. A large suction cup device is used to tent the skin up and the gas is injected. Advocates of the technique claim the recipient site (the butt) is optimized for allowing for the fat to live as an effect of the gas in the tissue. They claim there is better blood supply to the butt, and an increase in oxygen in the tissues. The people also claim tight spots are easier to inject into and the discomfort of the fat being injected is less. There are some that believe it is safer to inject with this technique, as more space is created in the tissue between the skin and the muscle.

I, personally, am not too impressed with this technique. The majority of these claims are antecdtocal and theoretical, and not backed by clinical science. Keep in mind, carboxytherapy (injecting Co2 gas under the skin) is used to break up tissue and dissolve fat to treat cellulite. This same gas now enhances fat retention in the butt? Not to mention, how long does the gas take to have these effects? Injecting the gas in the butt one time for a few hours I find hard to believe will have any real long term effects. From a results standpoint I have seen a few doctors work with it, and although it looks pretty cool while they are doing it, the results haven't impressed me more than a traditional result. If anything it is my belief it can give a doctor the false sense that an area is filled with fat when instead it is just bloated with the gas and swollen from the suction.

6. **Stromal Vascular Fractions**- are multiple types of cells (adipose-derived stem cells (ADSCs), mesenchymal and endothelial progenitor cells, leukocyte subtypes, lymphatic

cells, pericytes, and vascular smooth muscle cells) that are removed during liposuction. These cells have the potential to transform to other cell types to repair or rebuild tissue. They are being studied to be used as stem cell therapy. In the US the restrictions are very tight and therefore the potential is very limited. The use of the enzyme collagenase will help isolate these cells

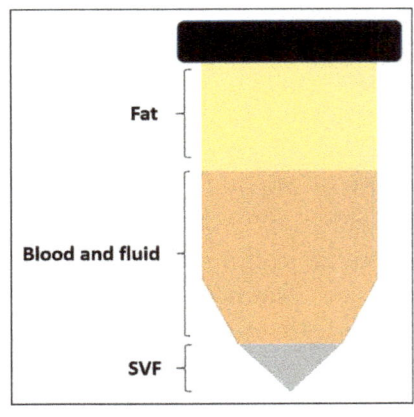

and because the lines between embryonic stem cells and these fat derived stem cells are blurry in the eyes of the FDA, limited clinical applications are being done in the US. Their belief is that fat is use to cushion and support tissue in the body and because it is coming out of the body, being manipulated and re-introduced for a potentially different purpose it falls under a different regulatory pathway. Isolating SVF for a Brazilian Butt lift is not really done because there are stromal vascular fractions that re being transferred along with the fat without needing to isolate them. They are responsible for the turnover of dying fat to new fat. They have been used in fat transfers to the breast to improve the very poor fat survival rate in fat transfer to the breasts. Currently the FDA only allows stem cell therapy from bone marrow and cord blood. The potential of fat is great. There is usually a large supply and it is much easier to acquire than other sources.

7. **<u>Threads for buttlifts</u>** - The desire of patients to get a better butt has made the butt business a booming industry.

Not every doctor is qualified to do a traditional Brazilian buttlift. Not every patient want to have surgery. When there is a patient who has money and the desire to spend it, you can bet your ass something will be used to take it; enter the thread world. Threads are temporary fixes and have been around for many years.

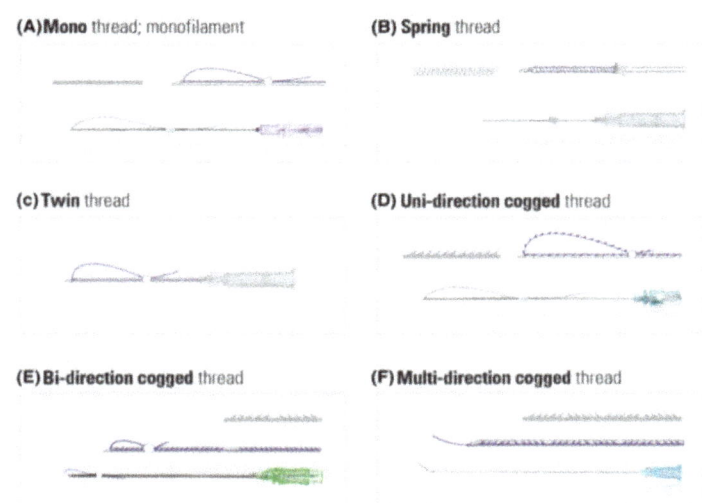

(A) **Mono** thread; monofilament

(B) **Spring** thread

(c) **Twin** thread

(D) **Uni-direction cogged** thread

(E) **Bi-direction cogged** thread

(F) **Multi-direction cogged** thread

There are different shaped threads with bards in different directions, and even dissolvable cones on the thread that help suspend the tissue. The three main types of materials used are polydioxanone (PDO), polylactic acid (PLA) and polycaprolactone (PCA). These are all dissolvable and last progressively longer in the order they were mentioned. These are ok in the face when done correctly and on the correct candidate. I do not believe they are appropriate for the butt.

The reason they work in the face is the skin they are pulling is much lighter than the volume in the butt. Additionally, this area is not under the same mechanical stresses as a butt that we use as a cushion all day long. In the face the the threads are used to pull the tissue back to anchorage points. In the butt, someone thought of a cool marketing idea calling this the spider butt lift with no true anchorage points. Instead a web of threads are created in the skin. Poking your ass with a needle 100 times and leaving a dissolvable thread under the skin will certainty cause swelling and inflammation that can hide minor depressions of the butt and even cause a *temporary* plumping.

Just like a person using their hands to stretch a wrinkle on a shirt you are wearing, these threads could potentially stretch out an irregularity to the skin as long as they are presently there. But there is no true lift here. Even if there was tissue being pulled up to a deeper stable point (which there is not), the tensile strength of these threads are not strong enough to lift the butt tissue. It would snap almost immediately.

I am not a believer in this. Oh what a tangled web we weave… you fill in the rest.

8 A quick Google search for enhancing your butt will bring on even more bullshit. Stay woke.

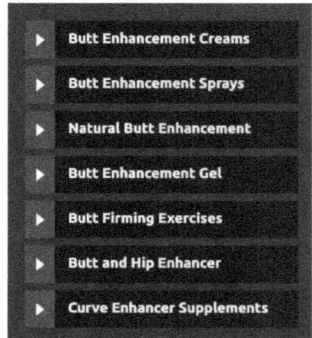

Chapter 41: Waist trainers

"Somethin' with a fly face, slim waist, big butt."
Trey Songz

Waist trainers are essentially a form of body modification that is not new but can dated back to sixteenth century Europe, most notably during the Victorian era. It has been worn most commonly under clothing but has also been worn as an outer garment as well. Fashion history reveals the first recorded corset originated from Crete in Greece, worn by the Minoan people. Both Minoan men and women wanted a small waist. As children, both genders wore a girdle around their waists that was tightened as they grew in order to stop growth in the waist area.

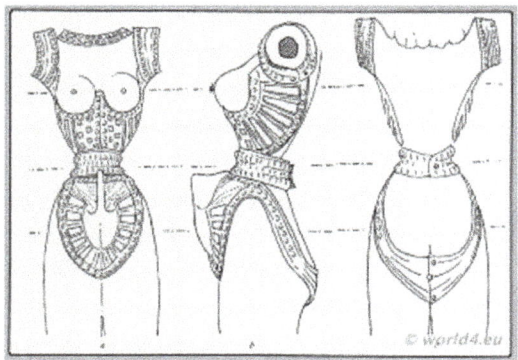 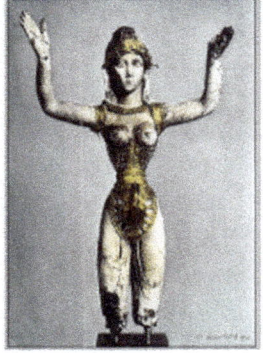

In the 1300s, bandages were used to slim the waistline under tight fitting clothes. At the end of the 1400s, front laces corsets were being used, enforced with strengthen fabrics or brass wires. Over centuries to come, the rich and famous of France, Spain, and England set the trends in what was worn in terms of waistline fashion. The styles evolved in terms of material used and design. Although the desired appearance of a smaller waistline remained the same, some corsets were more likely to enhance the breast area and waistlines shifted up and down.

In the US corset design was influenced by wartime constraints of materials combined with what was trending in Europe. Christian Dior, Jean Paul Gaultier, and icons such as Madonna kept the corset look en vogue in the US. Stars such as Beyonce, Shikara and Lady Gaga now wear corsets for their on-stage productions to add drama and femininity to their acts. And most recently, Kim Kardashian wears her's to train her body to alter her girlish dimensions.

Other cultures have used external forces and the body's response to these forces for many years.

Foot binding
From 970 AD to the 1950 about 3 billion women in China bound their feet to be trained to be smaller and pointy to attract men. This was done by wealthy women and essentially 50% of the Chinese women not allowing them to work in the fields.

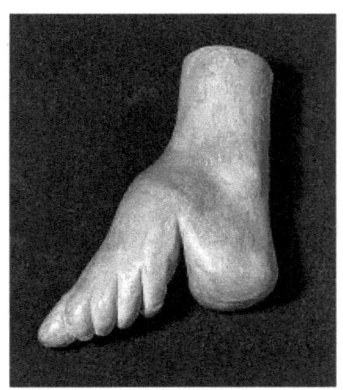

Starting at the age of 4-7 years old, young girls had their feet soaked in hot water mixed with animal blood for hours. The dead skin was scraped away and the nails were clipped and covered in talc. The soaked bandages would be applied by mom or an alderwoman in the village. Four toes would be tucked under and a figure 8 bandage breaking the toes would be performed so the heal becomes closer to the ball of the foot.

This manipulation of the foot continued until a final result of a deformed foot that looked like a 3 inch heel was achieved. These women could not walk. Foot binding was outlawed in 1912.

Neck elongating

For the past 1000 years, it has been customary in some Asian and African cultures to practice what is perceived to be neck elongation. Neck rings push the clavicle and ribs down. The weight of the rings twists the collarbone and eventually the upper ribs at an angle 45 degrees lower than what is natural, causing the illusion of an elongated neck. Because the rings have been on these women for such a long time, this weakens the neck muscles, rendering the neck essentially unable to support itself. The neck muscles will tire quickly and not be able to carry the weight of the head; in other words, when the neck is no longer able to fulfill its function it is very likely that it will collapse, thus resulting in suffocation.

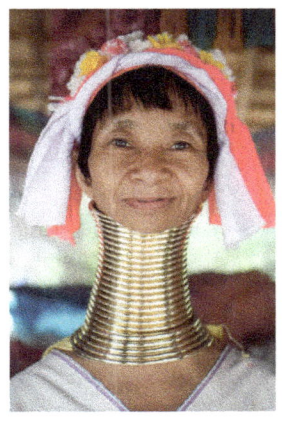

Ilizarov used external fixation devices on patients to treat non union of fractures in the 1950s. The apparatus is based on the principle which Ilizarov called "the theory of tensions". Through controlled and mechanically applied tension stress, Ilizarov was able to show that the bone and soft tissue can be made to regenerate in a reliable and reproducible manner.

Orthodontics
Another example of how consistent force applied to the body will promote change is in your mouth. Orthodontics, developed in the late 1800s, started using wires fixed to teeth by brackets to allow for teeth to shift to the shape of the bent wire.

"Medical experts" warn that wearing a waist trainer can cause heartburn, acid reflux, and make it difficult to breathe. These side effects develop from the waist trainer pushing a woman's stomach up into her diaphragm (MacMillan n.pag.). In addition, the waist trainer, can weaken a person's abdominal muscles. This causes permanent damage to their back, because they need those core muscles to support their spine (Kenway n.pag.). If a consumer wears the corset for longer than recommended, it can break their ribs, compress their lungs, and crush their organs (Thapoung n.pag.). According to Dr. Taz, "Your diaphragm, colon, liver stomach, and small intestines can all be shifted around inside your body after wearing one for too long" (Ross n.pag.). Women pass out from wearing the waist trainer for long periods of time so they can to get the results that the celebrities receive from "wearing" it. Doctors have confirmed that wearing a waist trainer, will only give women short term results, because the fat will eventually go back to where it came from (Thapoung n.pag.).

Other concerns according to the "experts" is these devices will:

- damage the liver
- decrease appetite
- decrease breathing

Most media outlets who have run a story about waist training condemns it. The points are essentially the same in all of the articles. For example,

ABC news recently published an article labeled, "4 Reasons to Throw Your Waist Trainer in the Trash". They shared their research in the following quotes:

"The Truth About Waist Training (and Why You Should Avoid it)
While wearing a shaping garment every now and then probably won't do any harm, long-term waist training is simply an ineffective way to slim down. It will do nothing to change your body proportions, and it can lead to many health problems. Here are just a few reasons why you should avoid waist training:

Waist training can damage vital organs
Remember that your torso is more than a column of fat and muscle—it's home to your lungs, stomach, liver, kidneys, and other essential organs. When you squeeze into a corset, these organs have to adapt, and they end up being pushed into unnatural positions where they are too crowded to function well. In the short-term, this likely just feels very uncomfortable, but long-term waist training can permanently harm organs, disfigure your body, or even fracture your ribs.

You will be slowly suffocating yourself
Waist training can deprive your body of oxygen, reducing lung capacity by an estimated 30-60% while you're wearing the corset. At best, this can result in low energy and discomfort, but scarier consequences—passing out, fluid buildup in the lungs, inflammation—are also a real possibility. Binding yourself in a

corset for weeks on end also restricts your lymphatic system, which relies on deep breathing and normal range of motion to properly remove waste products and toxins from your body.

You can cripple your digestive system
Your esophagus, stomach, and intestines form an intricate network in your abdomen, and extreme compression from a corset can hinder proper digestion. This can potentially cause blockages in your digestive tract, as well as give you acid reflux and other problems. Plus, any weight loss that does occur when wearing a waist trainer is likely due to the fact that your stomach is being crushed—and sacrificing your health for weight loss is simply a bad idea that will soon backfire. (In contrast, losing weight through making healthy changes will have many positive side effects.)

For all the females who think waist training is helping you become "skinny" 😒

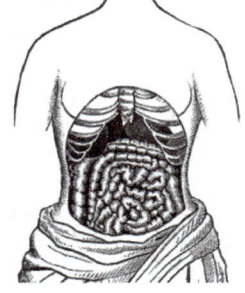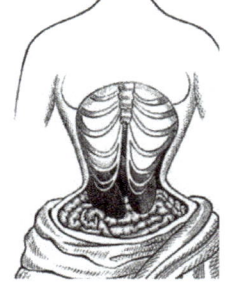

Waist training simply doesn't work
Contrary to what celebrities say, waist training will not reduce belly fat, make you lose weight, or give you similar results to liposuction. All a waist trainer can do is squeeze your torso for a temporary change in appearance. Like many get-thin-quick schemes, there is no evidence that weight loss while waist training is due to the corset rather than calorie restriction and exercise. In fact, the "health tips" from the Waist Gang Society, a vendor of waist trainers, states that "Wearing a waist-cinching corset, exercising and eating a healthy diet can radically reduce

your waist size." Even waist-training enthusiast Jessica Alba admits that diet and exercise were necessary to achieve her enviable figure. In other words, you can skip the pain, cost, and side effects of a waist trainer and simply focus on diet and exercise.

You cannot drastically change your body shape with a piece of fabric

Aside from losing weight, waist training is supposed to give you a perfect hourglass figure. The problem with this claim is that if hourglass curves are not your natural body shape, you simply are not going to have an hourglass shape once the corset comes off. Even the fittest of people have diverse body types and carry their weight differently; other than through surgery, you cannot dramatically change the shape of your body when you are already at a healthy weight.

The Beauty of Slimming Down Naturally & Proven Ways to Reshape

If you want to trim down and improve your body contours, there is no better method than adopting a healthy diet and exercising regularly. Watch your portions and swap out sugary, processed snacks for fresh, whole foods. Add strength training to boost your metabolism and tone muscles for a tighter tummy. A dietician, personal trainer, or physician can offer guidance on how to lose weight safely and suggest an exercise plan to help you reach your goals. Looking more vibrant and feeling happier are additional rewards you'll reap from healthy eating and regular exercise."

I think the confusion lies with medical experts and the media telling young impressionable women that it does nothing. If it does nothing, why is the next sentence a list of all the changes that take place within the body. Doctors are saying the only weight loss happens from sweating and by putting external pressure on your stomach decreasing appetite, but then says it's completely ineffective. Experts are sending mixed messages. Celebrities endorsing the product, and Instagram influencers, are saying that it is the answer to get the body they want.

This is what I believe to be true about waist trainers:
1. will decrease your appetite
2. immediately compresses and reposition your internal organs to a position higher inside of your body) (liver, intestines, lungs, diaphragm)
3. over time will reshape your liver, intestines, and ribs
4. will likely decrease fat over the areas it is cinching
5. it will likely decrease your core strength (abdominal muscles and back musculature)
6. it can decrease your blood return to your heart and your brain
7. short term it will do little to nothing to your figure.
8. long term it will change your body shape.

What does all of this mean?
1. eating less will cause weight loss
2. you can faint
3. altering the position of your internal organs can theoretically:
   a. cause constipation
   b. decrease your breathing capacity to more shallow breaths. This can cause a pneumonia
   c. your liver, and ribs will remodel to a constricted shape.

4. If blood return to the heart is compromised there is a a decrease in blood flow. As blood moves slower in theses 'kinked' areas, it is more likely to form a clot.
5. Does the body work less efficiently after these modifications? I am not sure.

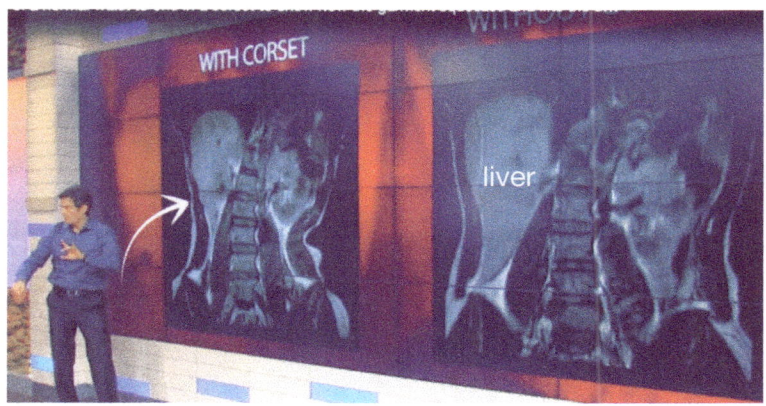

This is an image from the Dr Oz show, where they spoke to the dangers of waist training.

This is an MRI of a patient wearing a waist trainer on the left and without one on the right.
You can see the liver, intestines, and diagram are higher in the left image.
The arrow shows the ribs compressing into the liver.
It is obvious that the liver looks smaller in the picture on the left.

This is not from any studies I have performed but from basic scientific principles and articles I have read with regard to the subject.

Will wearing a waist trainer, purely by its physical pressure decreases fat around your midsection. While most medical professionals say no, my thoughts differ. Simply look at an elderly person who is bedridden. True, nutritionally they may be compromised, but many of these patients can get bedsores from sitting in the same position. These sores will erode through skin, fat, muscle down to bone if ignored. The power of a constant force on living tissue will cause the body to adapt. It is a basic theory of evolution. I do believe if worn for prolonged periods of time, waist trainers will decrease fat (not just because of a decrease in appetite), in addition to other changes discussed here.

In theory can these situations happen? Absolutely. Will it shorten or adversely affect your life? Theoretically. Is there any proof or is there a body of evidence showing people who wore waist trainers die before their time or have more health problems? None that I have been able to discover in hours of research in medical journals.

Doctors are always trained to be conservative and slow to adapt to trends so by reflex instinct they immediately condemn this practice because it is different. Their opinions are not based on sound research.

Do I believe waist training will decrease your waistline? Yes. Do I believe it is safe? I am not sure in the longterm. The only time I absolutely condemn waist training is after any abdominal surgery; whether it be a tummy tuck, liposuction, or any abdominal surgery. Your body needs to heal. Blood flow should not be restricted.

There are many factors at play here.
- The media loves a story that scares people.
- Doctors who many times don't know the answer need to have an answer and always will take the 'conservative' answer.

- Most celebrities will endorse anything for a price
- Most celebrities/instagram models modify their pictures. Their looks are how they make a living.

I share this information so you can make an educated decision. If it is was my daughter, I would not have her wear a waist trainer to modify her internal structure when the long term effects are no known. Especially because I want to be a grandfather one day (the effects are not known)! I am not condemning cosmetic surgery which modifies the external figure but worries about the consequences of modifying the internal workings of our organs. God laid out the body in such a way for us to function efficiently and I am not sure moving those parts around in a fixed space is a wise decision. Stay woke.

Chapter 42: The Art of the Twerk

Collaborative Author: The famous Ms. Gigi Maguire

Who am I?
I am Gigi Maguire, a superior entertainer, an illusionist and ... superhero. It's the way that I can fly across a stage, swing from pole to pole and fall from the ceiling to the ground so eloquently that will have anyone staring in amazement. I'm a woman of many talents!

Formally trained in dance, I was destined to entertain. Growing up in Philadelphia where I started dance classes since the early age of four, I became a well trained classical dancer. When life started getting the best of me and had backed me into a corner, I used what I knew how to do best to regain control of my situation. At 20 years old, I decided to enter the adult entertainment Industry as an exotic dancer.

Delilah's, Philadelphia's most prestigious gentleman's club, was the first club of my 10+ year journey as an exotic dancer. Something certain about me is that I always loved traveling. One weekend I took a trip to Atlanta for the first time and fell in love with the city. I came back to Philly with Atlanta on my mind. It took me five years to make the decision to leave my hometown but in 2005 I took the leap of faith and moved to Atlanta.

At the time I only knew one person in Atlanta, my cousin. I drove down to Atlanta with a friend from Philly who had been dancing in Atlanta already. I stayed with my cousin until I figured out my own place. I was in a new city and had to make some moves fast to get on my feet.

My friend was dancing at the world famous Magic City. Within the first couple of days I went with her to the club to check it out. I was going to apply to bartend there. She showed me around and introduced me to some of the girls who embraced me and were complimenting me all night. They assumed I was coming to dance there but I was done with dancing. I wanted to bartend now. Until one of them mentioned the amateur night contest on Wednesdays. I mean I wasn't there to dance but I could sure use the $500 cash prize. They had convinced me, so I entered... and won. Now I was ready to bartend there but the owner had other plans for me. Unbeknownst to me I actually made history that night as I was the first dancer that the Founder/Owner "Big Mag" had ever given an immediate offer to join the Magic City family. Although it wasn't my plan I figured, if he was impressed then I was looking forward to a good response from the customers.

While working at Magic City I met Fierce, another dancer whose style and presence undeniably matched my own perfectly, and soon after we became the first feature performers in the history of Magic City! (Second history making moment) The success of my exotic entertainment journey led to me become a staple at Magic City with people from all over the country traveling to Atlanta to see my illustrious performances.
I eventually supplied the demand of my audience by traveling all over the United States and to Canada as a feature performer along with a few fellow Magic City dancers. After some time Fierce, retired and moved on from dancing to the next chapter of her life. I had to find a new crew who had the same skills as me and luckily, I did. We became "The SnackPack."

Although I never sought out to be a model or video vixen, my reputation had people seeking me out to do both. I have been featured in several magazine spreads and music videos such as 2 Chainz & Nicki Minaj "Luv Dem Strippers," Jay Z's "Excuse Me Miss," Camron's "Oh Boy," Young Joc's "I Know You See It," and Trey Songz' "Brand new" and "Missing You" music videos, just to name a few.

In March of 2011, I expanded on my brand as Gigi Maguire and turned my love of dancing and seduction into a new business venture for me. I started my own company, PoleFanAddicts

Incorporated. PoleFanAddicts Inc. gave me the opportunity to share my talent and teach those who are interested in the art form a chance to learn from a true professional. I used pole dancing & twerk lessons as a form of fitness for my clients who wanted to get some tips but weren't interested in using it to be an entertainer. On the other hand for the girls already in the business or aspiring to be, I taught them new pole tricks, transitions and the art of seduction.

Shortly after starting Polefanaddicts, I transitioned out of dancing full time at Magic City to be able to put all of my focus into my business and teach full time. It wasn't long after building my clientele at the studio that I bid Magic City a farewell, but not without one last dance. See, I wasn't just your average dancer. It was the end of an era, for me and the club. It was only right that I gave my fans, friends and family one last time to see me perform on that legendary stage. So on December 12, 2011, I had my "Last Dance". (Third history making moment) I was the first dancer to "retire" and be celebrated for doing so.

Now... I'm here to teach YOU a few things.

When I first started dancing at Magic City I was amazed as to how the dancers moved. More specifically, how they shook their asses in a way that not only was hypnotizing but leaving me intrigued. HOW did they get each cheek to move the way it did with so much control AND rhythm. I needed to learn that skill. Yes, I could dance, and swing and FLY but I needed to get the hang of my butt like them! The way I learned was by watching. I watched and then mimicked what I saw and practiced. I practiced a lot. I was shaking, popping and working on my twerk all day, everyday. By any means necessary I was making my ass move... any time .. anywhere. While cooking, driving, or standing in line at the grocery store, seriously I was obsessed. Not only was I obsessed with making it twerk, I was also obsessed with making my cheeks jump one at a time. I was determined to make my little booty move they same way these big booty strippers were making theirs move!

One day I got up enough nerve to ask a fellow dancer how to do it and she explained it to me in a way that helped me figure it out.
Basically your booty muscle is the largest muscle in your body but it's also the weakest. We don't use it for anything except as a built-in seat cushion. Moving your booty muscle is all about control. In order to control the muscle you have to build it up and make it strong enough to be able to control it.

Squeezing and releasing the muscle almost the same way you squeeze when doing kegels. The first time I tried it I honestly was squeezing my thighs but as I kept trying I realized what muscle to squeeze and I went crazy with it. I squeezed and released my butt as much as I could until one day it happened!! I was able to make my cheeks jump one at a time. It was subtle at first, only little slight jumps, but as time went on and I kept doing it I eventually built up the muscle. Eventually it got strong enough that I'm able to make it jump significantly one cheek at a time. In my classes we refer to it as "One cheek, two cheek". I demonstrate and break down how to do it. Some of my students get it right away and some of them do as I did my first time trying and squeeze their thigh muscles, which is a great start actually. Eventually you learn the difference in the muscle and how to squeeze the right one. Now you try it.

Get down on the floor, sit up straight and spread your legs wide. Untuck your butt from under you as much as you can. Squeeze your right cheek and then your left cheek. Right cheek, then left cheek again, and again. You can start off slow to get your brain to connect with your butt and then when you get the hand of it, go faster. Now try it with some music. Tadaa!!! Now do that everyday until you gain some control and if you're not in the privacy of your own home, do the same movements at work at your desk, in the car, or on the line at the grocery store like I was!!!

When it comes to the traditional twerk there is a huge misconception that if you don't have a big booty then you can't twerk because there's nothing to move. I'm here to let you know that is not true. Anyone and everyone has the ability you just don't know how it works or how to make it work. But don't you fret.. I got you!
First thing you need to know is that it's your BODY not your BOOTY! If you move your body correctly the after effect will be the wiggle and jiggle of your booty ... no matter the size.
Another misconception is the way in which you are supposed to move. Now although there are plenty of ways to move and shake your booty there is also a science to the technique of how I personally teach it.

So... first things first.

Your stance. It's very important to stand with your feet at least shoulder width apart or wider but stay within your comfort zone. Poking out your chest and hips also helps.. in my class I refer to this as "put some stank on it!" It's in reference to the stank walk that you often see in the urban strip world. From there you want to keep your torso upright and bend the knees to get in your "drop it low" position.
Next comes another misconception and also where this "science" I spoke of is applied. Most women while attempting to twerk.. not only do they bend over at the hip they also bounce in the wrong direction, down! Bouncing in a downward motion is going with directional pull of gravity.
WRONG!
You want to bounce up so that gravity pulls you back down that way you get a different type of shake and wiggle in your booty. So bounce, Up Up Up Up Up Up Up Up... meanwhile in between, gravity does its job pulling it down. Simple right?

- Spread legs shoulder width apart
- Have a straight posture with your chest poked out
- Bend your knees only and drop down NOT bend over. (Like a squat)

- In the squatted position, bounce your butt UPWARD! If you need to hold on to your knees you can until you get the hang of it.

Next thing is the amount of force you put into those "Ups"! The more you move your body the more your booty will shake! The harder you go the more results you will see. You have to almost OVER do it to really get the maximum shake possible. Once you get into a good rhythm and you are comfortable with your twerk you can then try multiple ways of moving, such as in a circle. To achieve this you will simply rotate your hips while popping up.

You can also wiggle side to side almost like a doggie wagging it's tail. To achieve this you will start in your stance, feet at least hip width apart and don't forget to put the "Stank on it!" DO NOT BEND YOUR KNEES FOR THIS. From there you want to bend over at the waist and while keeping the butt muscles as relaxed as possible you just wiggle from side to side! Wag that tail like a happy lil puppy!!!

Lastly, you can also twerk on the floor on your hands and knees in the "doggy style" position. I'm this position you want you knees hip width apart, your hands placed right below your shoulders. In this position starting with a flat back you want to snap your hips up and your chest down simultaneously. Keeping in mind that the harder you move your body or "snap" the more your booty with shake. Down, up, down, up, down, up, starting slow until you feel comfortable enough to speed it up. This position is also good for twerking in a circle by simply moving your hips in a circular motion while you snap.

Some key pointers you always want to keep in mind is that you have to have the correct stance. Feet/knee placement is very important. The more you move your body the more your booty will shake. In order to control the butt muscle enough to make it pop you must build up the muscle to get strong enough to move it. Most importantly have fun with it and pass on what you've learned. Friends don't let friends, twerk wrong! Now turn on some music and practice, practice, practice.

I continue to entertain the masses with my talent as I've transitioned from one venture to the next while tangling them all in my web of greatness! I was featured on two episodes of "LaLa's Full Court Life" Season 2 on VH1. Lala Anthony is a dear friend of mine. She also mentioned me in her second book The Power Playbook in the same chapter of some great people like LL COOL J & Queen Latifah. I was also on "The Kandi Factory" on Bravo.

Personally, I have embarked on a whole new journey in life. I'm well known for changing the forecast but no one expected a modification like the one I made in October of 2013 when I decided to follow my heart and it led me to New York City. It had been 8 years since I lived on the northern east coast but you know the saying, "Love conquers all." Due to my major move to NYC, I decided to close my dance studio in Atlanta on January 31, 2014.
Upon my arrival to New York, I became a featured instructor at La Femme Suite in Harlem and Pole Basics in Philadelphia.

Apart from being a certified featured instructor, I toured as a celebrity host and featured performer all across the country until mid-2014. I worked as the Director of Entertainment at Vanity Grand of Philadelphia in 2015 from January until December. During my employment at Vanity Grand, I assisted in its transformation from a regular gentleman's club to a more upscale venue & event space.
In September of 2014, I added another title to my repertoire. I began my career as the co-host of the popular podcast, Angela Yee's "Lip Service."

If I must say so myself I have become a force to be reckoned with and I have no plans of letting up anytime soon. I'm on the rise to becoming an entertainment icon, a young female mogul if you will, so stay tuned for the rest of my successful voyage. I always has a few surprises up my sleeve, so we're sure the best is yet to come for Ms. Gigi Maguire!

I'm currently based in Atlanta and I teach by request only. Occasionally I have workshops and TwerkShop at various studios nationwide but I'm also available to be booked for private lessons or group parties. I am active on Instagram at @gigimaguire and for more information and rates for my services or appearances, by email at BookGigiMaguire@gmail.com

Ask. Believe. Receive.

Chapter 43: Excuses you can use if you wanna lie

"Only God can judge me."
                                        Tupac Shakur

I am all about honesty. If it was me I would tell the world I had a BBL done, however not everyone feels the same as I do. You have no obligation to tell anyone. However, be prepared to explain why your body looks so amazing after. I guess you can thank squats and fashionova jeans. But, explaining why you can't sit on a chair at work may be more difficult. Here are some excuses our patients have used and have been successful.

1. I had hemorrhoid surgery. Not the sexiest excuse in the book, but it will explain why you can't sit and why you need to sit with the special booty pillow (or boopy pillow)
2. I had a pilonidal cyst. Pilonidal cysts are caused by groups of hairs and debris trapped in the pores of the skin in the upper cleft of the buttock, forming an abscess. When I did my general surgery training, I had to drain a bunch of these. The smell is horrific. Again, this would not be my first choice of an excuse, but if you are willing to claim it, no one will question your dedication to the cover up cause.

3. I fell and broke my tailbone. Your coccyx bone is your tailbone what can be bruised or fractured with a fall on your butt. If fractured it can take 8-12 weeks to heal, so this certainly is a viable and most popular excuse.
4. I have bad sciatic pain and have relief when I sit on this pillow. Those with sciatic pain have a pillow that is similar in shape to the BBL pillow. I would just rip out the tag that says BBL pillow.
5. I had spinal fusion surgery.
6. I had surgery to treat Rectal prolapse. This is when part of the rectum protrudes from the anus. Maybe you want to avoid this excuse so you don't have to explain it to anyone.

Chapter 44: Haters

"I don't give a fuck. God sent me piss the world off."
                                                            Eminem

We all have haters. I got em, you got em. If you think you don't, look a little harder. They may have a smile on their face, but they are out there.

These are not all original thoughts of mine, but more of an amalgamation of things I've read, experienced, and thought about when pontificating.

Every living organism: a lady bug, a mouse, an elephant, a fish, an amoebae, a bacteria, and a human share one common want. We all have a desire to survive. We move towards things that help our survival. We sit close to those we like. On the flip side, we move away from pain. We fear things and distance ourselves to things that we see as a threat our survival.

I experience this in my profession from some of my colleagues because I am different from most of them. I have a busy operating schedule and a unique approach to communicating with my patients, and in their deep core, their animal instincts, they see me a threat to their survival. Whether they realize it or not they believe I am taking patients from them. I am taking away their livelihood, their ability to support their family, etc. I do not hate any of my colleagues without knowing them or having a real beef with them because I do not feel threatened by their success. There are so many patients for everyone, and there is a lid for every pot. If I became not busy for some reason, it will not likely be because others were doing better, I would look at myself as the problem and I would look to improve on a deficiency I may have. Not everyone has that type of mindset.

When you are looking better and having more confidence and posting fire pics on IG, your true ride or dies will be happy for you. Many others will call you lazy, fake, selfish, a thot, whatever the case may be. These are the people that actually fear you. They see you as threat to their success, happiness, and their survival.

Subconsciously, they are worried because you may be getting more attention than them. With more attention comes more interest from the opposite sex, more opportunities, more social engagements, more occasions to advance yourself- leaving them behind. The worst are the ones who you *think* are happy for you, but talk mad shit behind your back. It may take a while to discover these people are they often are a master of disguise.

I have seen women coming in for a surgery and they tell me their boyfriend is upset for getting the surgery and told her to just work out. Many times this falls under the same premise. They are fearful for *their own* survival. If you are looking fly and get more attention you may leave them, affecting them. Even I get a little crazy if I see my wife wearing someone a little too sexy to go to the gym herself. I trust her but I know there are a lot of guys who are animals.

Social media is interesting because now we have all these finsta[4] accounts that allow people to write whatever they want without any repercussions. It's a different world. I

---

[4] finsta is a fake instagram account

hate that side of social media. I can post a picture of a patient on IG that I think is dope and someone can write some stupid shit about it. It may hurt my feelings as an artist, and that's ok, I signed up for this shit. I feel worse for the patient who had the courage to have surgery and share their results with the world and now they are insulting them. It's kind of messed up.

Momma taught us two lessons that never reached this generation of social media jawns.

1. *Sticks and stones will break my bones but names will never hurt me.* Momma was full of shit with this one. To me, being called out on social media is horrible and it does hurt. I have raised money for and strongly stand against bullying. We have lost so many kids to suicide from being cyberbullied and many others live a life of depression as a result. I have seen patients in their 50s who still cry about things they were made fun of as a kid. If you are different you are seen as a threat to their survival.

2. *If you don't have anything nice to say, don't say anything at all.* Most people forgot this lesson all together.

Long story short. If you want to do this surgery, decide for yourself. I think guilt is a major factor for patients in not getting this surgery done when they really want it. Guilt in that maybe I am taking the easy way out and I could exercise, I can't spend the money, what if something happens to me, 'they' really don't want me to do it, what will 'they' think if i did it, 'they 'will be mad. If you are going to a reputable place and understand the risks, and have a way to pay for it without neglecting other important areas in your life it is simply a matter of another want. Fuck 'them'.

The best way to quite the haters and shut them down, is show them how you killin it. When they see you flexin and winning, they will slowly retract and retreat.

Chapter 45: FAQ

1. If i get lipo will my belly button look weird?

The only way your belly button will look weird after lipo is if you wear a garment that is too tight. Your belly button is not moved or altered in any way aside from a small incision to access the liposuction. Sometimes when the fat is removed around the belly button it can open ip a little. However, from the small incision inside the belly button it is possible to heal with a poor scar, just like any other area in your body.

2. How much does fat weight?

1 liter of fat = 2 pounds

3. How much downtime after surgery?

Everyone is different but we recommend you not sit for the first 10 days. Most of out patients we allow to resume work in 2 weeks, many choose to wait longer.

4. After the transfer what is the net amount of fat that will remain?

Everyone is different and lot has to do with aftercare, biology and the tightness of your butt. On the average most people retain at least 70% of the volume injected.

5. I have a heachache after surgery, what do I do?

The headache you are having after surgery is most likely due to dehydration. Try to drink much more than you regularly do. Your fluid requirements because of fluids lost, not eating or drinking before surgery, swelling, the stress of surgery causing a rise in cortisol levels, and bleeding all increases your requirements.

IF you are taking Percocet or Vicoden you cannot take Tylenol. These drugs all contain Acetominophen in it and you can overdose. Any type of buprofen is ok (Advil or Motrin), Aspirin (after day 3), Alleve, or Excederin is ok too. If this still does not work, a large glass of coffee usually does the trick.

6. Can I get 6 pack etching?

You certainly can however please be aware of these things. 6 pack etching looks nice on the table but:
a. I do not believe it is safe for the skin integrity during a tummy tuck
b. the areas that looks like 'muscle' is actually fat left behind and will feel soft
c. if you gain weight this fat areas will get bigger making you look like a waffle
d. the chance of seroma is at least 18% higher when it is done
e. you need to get many more massages after 6 pack etching
f. more incisions are often needed to get the horizontal lines across the muscle

I do 6 pack etching upon request but it is not for everyone. A lean person will look good. My personal taste is a woman looks nice with a line in the middle down, and the ones diagonally going to the groin. Horizontal 'cuts' look a little extra on women. On a dude that's lean it could look fire.

7. What is the maximum amount of fat that can safely be removed?

5 Liters. That is the law in many states like NY. Anything beyond that is called megaliposuction and has been associated with a higher rate of complications including death. 5 Liters is a lot of fat. This is what it looks like in Henney bottles.

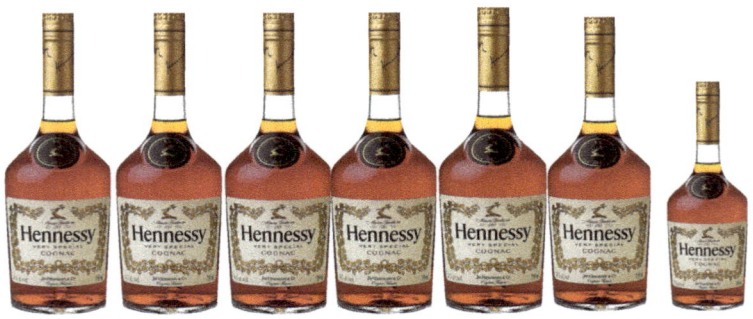

6. What is S.A.F.E. Liposuction?

S.A.F.E. was an acronym developed by plastic surgeon Dr. Simeon Wall. It stands for fat Separation, fat Aspiration, and Fat Equalization. The name **is not** to imply that this technique is a safer than other liposuction techniques and that other techniques are not safe.

Chapter 46: The future

"If no-one comes from the future to stop doing it, then how bad of a decision can it really be?"
Will Ferrell

The future of the BBL

I do not believe this is a fad that will go away and the fat booty is here to stay. I do however believe our technology will improve allowing us to get safer results and also legislation will follow Florida's lead putting more restrictions on this procedure.

Ultrasound is the only way I perform the BBL now. It is undoubtedly the safest way to inject fat and know where you are injecting it to avoid a fat embolism. I do believe it will become the standard of care in a matter of time.

There is a company that is developing an injection cannula that has a probe on the end that senses when you are in fat or in the muscle. It will actually shut down and not allow the injection to take place if it senses the cannula is in the muscle. This is not foolproof, as one an injury to the fascia covering the muscle is opened, you have created a pathway for the fat to get into the muscle. Filling the butt odeee or wearing a tight faja may propel the fat into the opening. Once it enters the muscular space as we mentioned in earlier chapters, the fat can seep through the muscle and sit next to the deep veins awaiting an injury which could be from manipulation only and not by cannula injury. Once that injury occurs the fat could be sucked into the vein and headed for problems. It is not infallible but it is a step in the right direction.

Many doctors are now becoming more conservative out of fear of injecting too deep, which is a great thing for safety but it could affect results. Will the patients tolerate a less than hoped for result? Before we knew of the dangers of muscular injections of fat many of us were getting lucky (apparently) and creating gorgeous projections on our BBLS. A very superficial fat transfer to the butt will create little to no projection. To get my projection I inject under Scarpas fascia and over the muscle with my ultrasound so I can safely go deep. Even with that, sometimes patients want more projection or their butt, but the skin is so tight it will not stretch outward. For these people, a composite BBL, or hybrid BBL, or super charged BBL (chose your adjective) may be considered. I do believe they will become more popular in the years to come and they are just starting to be done more now.

I cover this in more depth in the chapter about silicone implants. To summarize the concept it is a small implant for some bulk placed deep IN the muscle, surrounded by fat over the muscle to make the butt more shapely and soft. It is a combine approach to get the best of both worlds.

As the popularity of having a fat ass continues to grow, and as the media continues to focus on the fears and dangers of this procedure more non surgical alternative will continue to arrive. With that there will be more bullshit techniques, creams, devices, threads, injections, drinks, garments, lasers (you name it) to try to capitalize on this multi-billion dollar market. Everyone will claim to be an ass making expert. New alternatives in fillers will continue to come to the market. Already there are fillers used in Europe that have not yet been released to the US for this enhancement procedure.

In the very near future we anticipate the release of CoolTone, made by Allergan (the makers of Botox, Juvederm, CoolSculpting etc). Additionally TrueSculpt Flex is another new device in this new category. These machines are intended to help strengthen and tone muscles. It does this via magnetic muscle stimulation (MMS), which basically fires electromagnetic energy into your muscles to cause involuntary contractions. Like a TENS unit. The body's response to these involuntary contractions is to strengthen the muscle fibers underneath the targeted area of treatment. The result is supposedly stronger, firmer, and more defined muscles. This is similar to Emsculpt, already on the market. The cost for the CoolTone and TrueSculpt Flex devices are significantly less for the physician to purchase therefore we expect the treatments to cost less, and potentially this will drive down the cost of Emsculpt as well.

As I mentioned in earlier chapters the use of an ultrasound device during BBL injections will save lives and it is a matter of time before it becomes the standard of care, and maybe even turned into legislation. I believe as more surgeons become educated about newer research the need for unnecessary hospital admissions and blood transfusions will decrease as the use of transexemic acid becomes more popular and cell savers start to find their way in office based surgical suites.

The World Association of Gluteal Surgeons (WAGS) is a multidisciplinary organization who's sole purpose is to educate doctors on how to make the BBL safer, and to inform patients allowing them to make good decisions on their care. It started in a group text between myself, Dr. Miami, and few other doctors in our squad. We were discussing some of the deaths that had occurred in the news from the procedure and heard of the threats for putting an end to this surgery. I mentioned that the "BBL needs a rebranding- a good publicist". Dr. Miami and his team then took action to create this group that now encompasses 35 countries and about 200 doctors; growing by the week. We are creating better guidelines, safe protocols, and a more accurate estimations on how prevalent a problem this is. We have been successful in helping guide legislation in Florida for this procedure and had our first summit in early 2020.

Real self is a website many of our patients are familiar with. One of the features of this site is a section where patients can pose questions and multiple doctors will answer them. No matter what the question is, all the responses for BBL concerns contain at least (and sometimes only!) the tag line "make sure you consult with a Board Certified Plastic Surgeon". Sometimes the question hasn't even been answered, it is like an automated robotic response to any concern a patient has. The truth is, Board Certified Plastic Surgeons along with other non Board Certified Plastic Surgeons are killing patients with this procedure. Being a Board Certified Plastic Surgeon has not shown to have less deaths from a BBL than any other surgeon performing this surgery. I know Board Certified Plastic Surgeons that has never been taught and never done a BBL before. Education in this surgery needs to be through continuing education, taking courses, endless reading and learning, and mentorships. No surgeon or group of surgeons can sit on their high horse and believe they are shielded from this. Patients are dying from this elective procedure. Taking this surgery away is not the answer. Patients will go to other countries or less qualified doctors where they may be even more at risk for a complication. WAGS is a huge step in the right direction where doctors act like colleagues rather than competitors all working together for a common mission to protect our patients that have put their trust in us.

About the author:

Dr. Scott Blyer, aka DrBfixin, is in private practice in Long Island, NY. He has become quite famous for his unique style and his body transformations, most notably his BBL surgeries. He has performed thousands of such surgeries safely in his office based surgery center. He lives in NY with his wife, daughter, and his two dogs (Chloe and Daisy). Although Dr Blyer has published many peer reviewed articles in medical journals and text books, lectured on the BBL, this is his first type of project to the general public. He has a very active instagram page and snapchat account where he teaches, entertains, and shows his surgeries and his results. His Tiktok account is just for clowning around.

If you are interested in a consultation to discuss the possibilities towards your dream body you can:
1. call the office for a consult 631 232 2636
2. sign up for a online/virtual Skype or Facetime consultation Drbfixin.com
3. or email drb@cameosurgery.com with your contact info

Thanks for reading this book. I am quite proud of it. It took a while to put together and I truly hope it will help you in your journey and keep you out of harm's way.
On to the next project.
Always Bfixin 🔧,

Dr. Scott M Blyer

Instagram @DrBfixin
Snapchat @DrBfixin
TikTok @Dr.Bfixin
Facebook @CameoSurgery

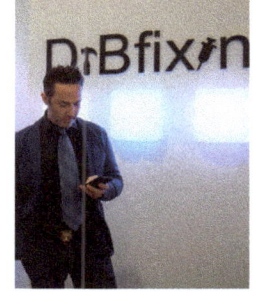

www.ingramcontent.com/pod-product-compliance
Lightning Source LLC
Chambersburg PA
CBHW042113100526
44587CB00025B/4030